Factors Influencing the Implementation of The Care Programme Approach

A research study
carried out for the Department of Health
by Social and Community Planning Research

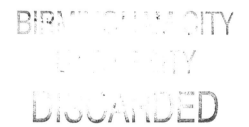

Cathy North   Jane Ritchie

Kit Ward

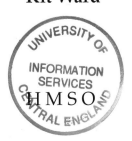

HMSO

Contents

Acknowledgements

This research was undertaken by Social and Community Planning Research, on behalf of the Department of Health. We would like to thank Elisabeth Parker, David Kingdon, Mary Hancock, and Glyn Lewis from the Department of Health for their guidance and support throughout the study.

The evidence in this report is derived from the views and experiences of staff from health authorities, social services departments and voluntary agencies, as well as service users and their carers. We are grateful to them all for the time and thought they gave to the discussions and for the openness with which they responded. This contributed greatly to the learning gained from the research.

Foreword

Mental illness, once dubbed the Cinderella of the National Health Service, is now moving into the limelight. It is designated one of the five key areas requiring particular attention in the Government's strategy "The Health of the Nation". The Government is committed "to improving the health and social functioning of mentally ill people" and to effecting a significant reduction in the rates of suicide. The Care Programme Approach is the co-ordinated therapeutic action which is essential to achieving these aims.

The Approach is based on best professional practice and provides for the systematic assessment of both health and social care needs of mentally ill people and a key worker whose duties are to keep in close touch with the patient and monitor that the agreed plan of care is delivered. It is these means which will help to ensure that severely mentally ill people do not fall through the network of care.

This report explores in depth how the Care Programme Approach is being implemented in four district health authorities with very different characteristics and discusses the many issues involved in its implementation. The progress made so far by the districts is described in a way that is helpful to others, and the difficulties are not glossed over. It will assist managers and mental health teams by highlighting both the practical problems that provider units will need to overcome and by providing examples of solutions to those problems.

This report by SCPR joins the Mental Illness Key Area Handbook as essential reading for anyone involved in the planning, purchasing and delivery of mental health services. I commend it to you.

CHIEF MEDICAL OFFICER   March 1993
Department of Health

PART I

THE IMPLEMENTATION OF THE CARE PROGRAMME APPROACH

CHAPTER 1 Introduction

1.1 Background

The care programme approach (CPA) for people referred to specialist psychiatric services was implemented in April 1991. The approach requires district health authorities, in collaboration with social services departments, to design and implement systematic arrangements for deciding whether a patient can be treated in the community and, if so, ensuring that they receive the necessary health and social care. Each district health authority, in conjunction with the relevant social services department/s, determines the form that the care programme approach will take in their local area.

The Department of Health Circular HC(90)23 states that all care programmes should include the following elements;

i.   Systematic arrangements for assessing the health care needs of patients who could, potentially, be treated in the community, and for regularly reviewing the health care needs of those being treated in the community.

ii. Systematic arrangements, agreed with appropriate social services authorities, for assessing and regularly reviewing what social care such patients need to give them the opportunity of benefitting from treatment in the community.

iii. Effective systems for ensuring that agreed health and, where necessary, social care services are provided to those patients who can be treated in the community.

The Circular emphasises the importance of inter-professional collaboration, both within the health service and between health and social service professionals. It also stresses the need to involve patients and carers in discussions about proposed care programmes.

In 1991, the Department of Health commissioned a research study to examine the implementation of the care programme approach. This report presents the findings of the study. The research was carried out between August 1991, a few months after the planned start of the care programme approach, and October 1992.

1.2 Objectives of the Study

The central aims of the study were to examine how the care programme approach is being operated in different authorities and the factors that are contributing to, or inhibiting, its effective implementation.

To do this the study has investigated;

-   The policies that were developed to deliver CPA and the extent to which these were successfully implemented.

- The procedures that were introduced to implement CPA and how effective these have been in practice.

- The extent to which the principles of CPA have been adopted and the changes in aftercare planning and delivery that have resulted.

The results of the study are intended for use by both the Department of Health and by individual health and social service authorities to identify areas where guidance or intervention in the implementation of the CPA is needed.

It should be noted that the aims of the research have had to be modified as the work progressed. It was originally intended that the study would have a more focused objective in helping to determine some of the *outcomes* of introducing the care programme approach. In particular, the Department was concerned to know more about the numbers and characteristics of patients who were offered treatment only on an in-patient basis because of a failure to provide appropriate care in the community - and the reasons that led to this. In the event, it was not possible to meet these objectives because the implementation of the care programme approach, and, in particular, its monitoring, was not sufficiently advanced in any of the authorities studied to allow these specific factors to be judged. The reasons for this are more fully discussed in the later sections of the report.

1.3   Design and Conduct of the Study

A staged programme

It was initially intended that the research should be carried out in one phase in the latter part of 1991. This plan assumed that the care programme approach would be fully implemented in health authorities by the autumn of 1991. Preliminary investigation showed that, while planning for the implementation of CPA had taken place in all districts by then, it was still very much at an evolutionary stage. There were still discussions ongoing about how CPA should be defined and operated within the authorities and there were still details of implementation to be resolved.

In view of this, it was felt to be premature to undertake the full programme of research at that time. There was a danger that the research would simply identify aspects of CPA implementation that were subject to piloting and change. It was therefore agreed with the Department that a phased programme of work should be undertaken.

The first phase, carried out between August and November 1991, investigated the planning and design of CPA in each area, and the issues that were raised by its implementation. It also identified any monitoring systems that were being put into place. An interim report on this stage was submitted to the Department of Health in January 1992.

The second phase, carried out between April and October 1992, investigated the operation of the CPA at working level, with the principal aim of identifying factors that aid or inhibit its full implementation.

The study areas

The research was undertaken in four health authorities. These were selected by the Department of Health to provide diversity in terms of geographical location, co-terminosity with social services departments (SSDs), type of catchment area and history of psychiatric services (Section 1.4). The related social services departments (seven) were also approached and all took part in the research.

Method of investigation

The research was designed to be exploratory and investigative in form so that it could be responsive to the events occurring in each authority. Unstructured, interactive interviews were used to collect information from those participating so that the issues raised by different participants could be explored. The interviews were based on broad topic guides which outlined the key areas for discussion (see Appendix B). The interviews were all tape recorded so that there was a verbatim record of each for analysis.

Over the two stages of the research, interviews were carried out among a number of different professionals. These included:

-    health and social service managers

-    development officers in charge of implementing CPA

-    consultant psychiatrists and hospital doctors

-    ward managers and nurses

-    social workers (both hospital and community based)

-    occupational therapists

-    community psychiatric nurses

-    clinical psychologists

In addition, interviews were held with a small number of patients and carers and with members of local voluntary agencies.

The focus at the first phase was on those who had been involved in determining CPA policy and preparing for its implementation. Thus, the majority of those interviewed were members of working groups and were mainly at management level within their professions (for example nurse managers, operational managers, social work team leaders, and heads of occupational therapy or clinical psychology departments). A number of consultants were also interviewed, although they were not all closely involved in CPA planning.

At the second stage greater emphasis was placed on staff involved with CPA on a daily operational level (eg CPNs, social workers, ward staff, occupational therapists etc). Further consultations also took place with key individuals who were involved in the first stage. Also, at the second stage, the interviews took place with ex-patients, carers and members of local voluntary agencies.

A total of 169 people were interviewed in the course of the study, of whom 33 were interviewed on two or more occasions. Further details of the number and coverage of the different groups consulted are shown in Appendix A.

A systematic analysis of the information collected was carried out using a broad thematic framework. This made it possible to compare and contrast policy, practices and experiences, both within and between the four study areas. This in turn led to the identification of key factors that either facilitated, or hindered, the full implementation of the care programme approach.

1.4   A Profile of the Study Areas

A brief description of the areas is needed in order to place the study findings in some context. There is, however, a difficulty in providing descriptions since it was agreed that the identity of the four areas should remain unknown. This was to encourage an openness of response in the investigations as it was recognised that the issues faced by these authorities would be mirrored in many other authorities. The profile of the areas is therefore presented in general terms so as to prevent identification. The purpose of the profile is to highlight key differences between the authorities since these underlay the basis of their selection.

Geographical location and catchment area

The authorities were based in four different health regions covering areas in the east Midlands, west Midlands, the north of England and London. The catchment areas included both inner and outer city areas of high density population, smaller urban communities and rural areas. Two of the authorities serviced communities with relatively high proportions of people from ethnic minority groups.

Two of the authorities had catchment areas that were co-terminous with the local social service departments. In the other two, catchment areas covered more than one local authority area and hence two or three social service departments were involved with community care programmes.

Hospital services

Two of the authorities were responsible for large specialist psychiatric hospitals. Each of these was in the process of being closed, although there were still sizeable numbers of patients in residence.

All of the authorities had responsibility for large general hospitals which had psychiatric units. These contained acute, rehabilitation (or resettlement) wards, wards for elderly people with mental illness and out-patients' departments. There were also specialist units based within the hospitals such as intensive care units, resettlement units, mother and baby units and child and adolescent teams. In two areas individual acute wards admitted patients from specified geographical sectors of the community while in the other two sectorisation was not a feature.

Acute wards were generally far busier than rehabilitation facilities, having a high turnover of patients. Patients in acute wards were also more diverse in terms of their illnesses and needs. For these reasons, existing practice concerning discharge and aftercare was more advanced and comprehensive for rehabilitation or resettlement patients. In all four study areas, procedures had been developed in the rehabilitation facilities which already met many requirements of CPA. Major contributing factors here had been the lower turnover of patients and a greater amount of staff time available to invest in planning and implementing aftercare.

Community Health Services

In two areas, community mental health teams had been established. These were joint ventures incorporating staff from both health and social services. The composition of the teams varied but four or five disciplines were commonly represented, for example consultants, CPNs, social workers, occupational therapists and clinical psychologists. The teams served specific geographical sectors of population and were based in the community within their catchment area. In the other areas, CPNs and social workers were organised into separate teams related to specific geographical areas.

A number of specialist community based teams had also been established. These were often aimed at a defined client group, for example elderly people or people being resettled from long stay hospitals.

Day hospital facilities were provided by each of the health authorities. Sometimes these were for specific groups such as the elderly. Day centres were run by either health or social services and, in some cases, jointly. A variety of group and individual activities were offered within these settings.

Social Services Provision

Social services departments were not always organised in such a way that services for people with mental illness came under the remit of one designated manager. In one area, for example, responsibility was allocated by geographical sector rather than client group.

In all four areas the social services departments provided a range of residential care establishments for people with mental illness, most of which were staffed to some degree. They also played a key role in the provision of day care.

All of the social services departments employed a number of social workers to work with people with mental illness. On the whole, these were specialist posts devoted to mental health. In one area, however, mental health social work services were provided by generic social workers, although this was about to change.

All areas had hospital based social workers, who often worked as part of consultant led teams. Others worked in community teams, either jointly with health authority staff or solely led by social services. Social workers were also often involved in, or responsible for, specialist teams such as mother and baby units, resettlement teams and care management teams.

Relationship between HAs and SSDs

Relationships between the health authorities and their corresponding social services departments varied both between and within study areas. In two areas, for example, there were very good relationships at ground level, while at strategic level joint planning was not strongly established. Where there was more than one social services department involved with the health authority, relationships with each varied for both historical and other reasons.

In all areas there were established forums for discussion between health authority and social services department staff at different levels of seniority. The effectiveness of such forums varied.

Voluntary Sector

The voluntary sector was active in each study area, principally with the involvement of MIND and the National Schizophrenia Fellowship (NSF). There were commonly strong inter-relationships between the statutory and voluntary sector, with health authority and social services department staff playing key roles on the committees of the voluntary organisations. The degree to which voluntary organisations were consulted about health authority and social services planning varied (see Chapter 3).

1.5 Structure of the Report

The remaining chapters of this report summarise the main issues that arose during the development and early implementation of the care programme approach. Part I sets the scene by describing how CPA is viewed in terms of its perceived aims and advantages and how it was planned and developed in the four study authorities. Part II then considers how CPA has been operated in practice and the implications it has had for both staff and patients. Part III draws together the evidence collected and considers areas where future work might be targeted.

The evidence collected is set out in thematic, rather than area specific, form so as to highlight the issues involved. The anonymity of the individual interviewees who took part in the study, as well as the areas, is preserved.

CHAPTER 2 The Principles of the Care Programme Approach

2.1 The key Features of the Care Programme Approach

The central requirements

The care programme approach was introduced to improve the adequacy of arrangements for the care and treatment of people with mental illness in the community. Its purpose is to ensure that patients treated in the community receive the health and social care they need. The intention is to apply CPA to *all* patients referred to specialist psychiatric services so that no patient who might be vulnerable is missed.

The joint circular to health and social services authorities introducing CPA specified some requirements to achieve its basic aims;

- Systematic arrangements for assessing the health and social care needs of patients who could be treated in the community.

- Effective systems for ensuring that agreed health and social care services are provided to patients who can be treated in the community.

- Systematic arrangements for reviewing the health care and social care needs of those being treated in the community.

- Where a patient's minimum health or social care needs for treatment in the community cannot be met, in-patient treatment should be offered or continued.

Local implementation

The DoH circular specified that individual health authorities, in discussion with social services departments, should agree the exact form that the CPA should take and establish suitable local arrangements to implement it. It was specified that, in determining such arrangements, proper attention should be given to certain features of required practice.

Those highlighted were;

- Inter-professional working.

- The involvement of patients and carers.

- Mechanisms for keeping contact with patients being treated in the community, specifically though key workers.

Resources

Health authorities were expected to meet any costs arising from the introduction of CPA procedures from within existing resources.

However, the DoH circular stated clearly that the CPA placed no new requirement to provide services on either health or social services authorities. It was for health authorities to judge 'what resources they make available for such services' in the light of previous guidance. Social services authorities were asked to make similar decisions, although attention was drawn to the mental illness specific grant which was available from 1991/92 to increase the social care available for people with a mental illness.

It was stated in the Annex to the circular that decisions concerning the provision of community care or treatment for individual patients needed to take account of the resources currently available. If the lack of resources prevented acceptable arrangements bring made then, with the patient's consent, in-patient treatment should be offered or continued.

The elements summarised above comprise the essential features of CPA. The following sections of this report will consider how these were interpreted and implemented. Before embarking on discussion of the operational aspects of CPA, it is important to consider how the basic principles of the initiative were viewed.

2.2 Views on the Principles of the Care Programme Approach

At the first stage of the study, when CPA was initially being introduced, there were mixed views about the principles and features it embodied. On the positive side there was generally widespread agreement that the concept embraced important aspects of good practice, and that its introduction would help to formalise these. In particular, it was felt that CPA would help to ensure more systematic assessment of patients needs, would improve the quality of discharge planning and aftercare provision and would prevent patients *'falling through the net'*. It was also felt, by some professionals, that the process of operating CPA would help to enhance inter-agency and multi-disciplinary working, would encourage a more client centred approach, and would promote greater accountability among professionals for patients' aftercare. A particular benefit in the longer term was the potential of CPA to identify missing resources.

There was equally some resistance to the principles of CPA at the outset. Of prime concern, particularly to consultants, was the perceived impingement on clinical practice and judgement. There was also some resentment of what was seen as a government imposed procedure when the basic requirements of 'good practice' were already felt to be in place. But by far the major criticism from all groups of professionals was of the 'bureaucratic' and over-structured procedures that CPA was seen to require.

By the second stage of the study, when CPA was being more fully implemented, there had been some shifts in view. Although, for some professionals, the realities of CPA had simply confirmed their original opinion, others were modifying their appraisal - both positively and negatively - of its basic features. However, the key issues around which the debate occurred remained largely unchanged, with the following features attracting the most comment.

Systematic procedures

The basic intention of CPA to provide more systematic procedures for the assessment, planning and delivery of patient care was generally welcomed by all groups of professionals, particularly non-medical staff. Most were of the view that anything that helped to ensure that patients' needs were not overlooked or that individual patients did not get lost in the system was beneficial.

> "...through our forms we sit down and think, 'Well, what do we need for this person in terms of actioning community care?'. So that dialogue is taking place...in certain cases it obviously used to (happen) but it is part and parcel of the process." (Health service manager)

> "I think it's made me think a bit more systematically about aftercare and to go about it in a more methodical way...yes, I would say that." (Consultant psychiatrist)

> "I thought the whole idea of discharge and aftercare was a very positive thing and it made so much sense in that the management of a client's case could truly become multi-disciplinary and that there would be more active planning. I still think it provides the mechanism for that, it's a super attempt...it moves away from the old idiosyncratic way of psychiatric treatment to a much more structured, systematic approach to client care" (Clinical psychologist)

> "I think that what the care programme approach does, in creating this sort of system, it has become more systematised in its way of looking at what we need to do for which of the patients" (Health service manager)

> "I think discharge plans tended to be very hit and miss depending on how attentive the ward staff were and how good communication was with the community services, whereas now, hopefully, those loopholes that were there will be stopped." (Occupational therapist)

Although there was little dissent about this as a positive feature of CPA, there were some professionals who felt that such procedures were already in place. This view was mainly expressed by resettlement or rehabilitation teams.

> "We already had a system and when we saw the care programme approach we looked at it and thought there is nothing in this that we are not already doing . In fact we are doing more." (Health service manager)

Universal application

There was criticism that the requirement to apply CPA to all patients was unnecessary. In particular it was felt that the procedures associated with CPA were extremely over elaborate for the needs of many patients. This, accompanied by the paperwork requirements of CPA, led to the view that CPA was mistaken in its universal concept.

> "I personally feel that if the government had just introduced it in selected cases it would have been useful. By making it open for all cases the whole programme is frustrating, it has diluted the efficacy of it and all that it has done is for people to say 'I've got such a big work load'" (Consultant psychiatrist)

> "...I think it's unrealistic to expect us to have a written aftercare plan and three monthly review meetings for everyone who goes through. I don't see how we can do that without taking up a vast amount of our time." (Consultant psychiatrist)

Although the comments above came from consultants, there were other professionals who were equally critical of the requirement to include everyone. Indeed, as is examined later, this had led some authorities to make CPA selective in practice, even if, in theory, it applied to all patients (see Chapter 4).

Accountability

There was a hope on the part of some professionals that CPA would improve professional accountability for people with severe or continuing care needs. CPA had the potential to ensure that lines of responsibility for provision - both within the different authorities and between professional groups - were clear.

> "It will (make a difference), especially if it is brought in as a legal requirement. People are having to be more responsible ... taking responsibility for making sure that a person gets what they need." (Occupational therapist)

> "I think that what CPA has done is to make people more acutely aware of the kind of things they have to be arranging for people, and it is making them more aware of the potential complexity of discharging someone and how imperative it is going to be in the future for us and the local authority to plan jointly together to make sure that the kind of services that are needed for people in this unit allows them to be discharged" (Health service manager)

Identifying gaps in resources

> "...if the idea is to make sure that people aren't lost to the services and to identify unmet needs due to lack of service provision, I think that is wonderful." (CPN)

"I think the care planning process is going to change the world so to speak as far as community provision is concerned...If you can't supply what is in the care plan, sooner or later somebody is going to say 'Why does this keep coming up? How can we better supply it?'" (Health service manager)

The potential of CPA to monitor and identify gaps in services was a feature that was understood and widely acclaimed. Alongside this, however, there was considerable scepticism about whether such information would come to light and, more significantly, what would be done about it if it did.

The need for resources to implement CPA

There was consistent criticism that it was unrealistic of the government to introduce CPA without additional resources. These criticisms focused on two aspects. First, that the introduction of new procedures for care programming in itself required extra staff time -both at strategic and operational level. Second, many professionals argued that it was abundantly clear already that additional resources were needed to provide effective community care and that the introduction of CPA should have been accompanied by some recognition of this.

"I think the care programme approach is about providing good practice and if it does that's fine - it may be uncomfortable to have some criticisms and faults pointed out but if that is in the interests of a better service, then you put up with that... On the other hand, if it doesn't actually enhance the service but detracts from it by taking away some time, then that's a bad thing...I think it has used resources. You can say that starting something up does take resources and the benefit will come later, but I'm not too sure it will do anything more than balance even. I can't see it in this service which I think runs reasonably well, I don't think it is that necessary..."
(Consultant psychiatrist)

"I have no problem at all with the concepts behind the care programme approach and care management and I know we are not supposed to say we don't have enough resources - throw more money at it - but if you have a very low level of resources, changes in the concept and the model can only help so far. There is a lower limit and if you drop below that in terms of resources, basically you are just improving your co-ordination of a vacuum, and it's not terribly helpful." (Health service manager)

"We are totally underprovided with the basic bread and butter things that you need to run a mental health service - and that applies to social services and the health side...Its all very well to have a top heavy assessment thing as in our case, to have detailed planning, its not going to actually mean anything in practice. We have to have the systems that are going to deliver care. That's what is painfully lacking round here...the systems for delivering care are pathetically inadequate." (Consultant psychiatrist)

"The care programme approach is seen as something that is going to have to be done properly at some point or other. People see that there is a good

reason for it to be happening but they just wish there were enough resources." (Occupational therapist)

"My gut reaction was, 'Yes, its a jolly good idea but who is going to put resources into it?' and that is still the way I feel. There are a lot of really committed people out there, trying to do more than they are paid to do and it's still not enough and they know that…but right down the line, everybody -social services, housing, health authority, ourselves…everybody is asked to do a job which they are not being resourced for." (Voluntary agency)

Tackling problems at the wrong level

There was a view among a few professionals that the introduction of the care programme approach was simply tackling problems at the wrong level. This, in part, arose from the view above that the real issue was the lack of adequate resources for mental health services. It also arose from a feeling that CPA had been introduced as a compensatory measure for areas of bad practice, some of which had attracted significant public attention. It was argued that the latter problem would have been better tackled by targeted measures, rather than imposed procedures on the whole service.

"What the government could have done, with the doctors starting an audit system, they could have used the audit commission as a way of ensuring proper care, rather than this type of statutory obligation for a multi disciplinary team. It is taking a lot of our time un-necessarily to the point that we are writing things up that we are not looking at …" (Consultant psychiatrist)

"CPA is just the fine tuning - the bit that has got to be got right is developing a shared culture about who comes into hospital and who doesn't and why, and who priority groups are and what sort of hospital provisions you need for them. Until you have done all that, a CPA which deals with it long after this has happened is not going to be able to do anything else except ratify the mess that is already there. Like a lot of other governmental reforms (eg quality assurance and clinical audit) they are not tackling the real issues" (Social services manager)

"CPA assumed that the service was likely to be uniformly bad and rather than taking severe action in the bad places where people were being given 12 week appointments rather than being seen in the same week. It tried to supply the a solution - told us how to spend our resources - when we might have been able to spend them in a better way. It's an excellent, noble, laudable idea but it is not achieved by setting up a uniform system to cover the whole country -it is achieved by having the individual hospital units working efficiently and not being overstretched." (Consultant psychiatrist)

The patients interviewed were mostly not aware of CPA as either a Government or health authority policy. When the principles were explained to them reactions were usually positive. There was some scepticism, however, that in reality CPA would not work properly or would amount to paying lip service to care planning, rather than making any real difference.

2.3 *The Relationship Between CPA and Care Management*

Assessment and care management were initiatives set out in the white paper "Caring for People". Procedures were to be fully implemented by April 1993 with social services taking the lead. The Department of Health Policy Guidance "Community Care in the Next Decade and Beyond" (HMSO, 1990) defines care management as follows;

> "...care management in its most comprehensive form covers three distinct processes:
>
> - assessment of the user's circumstances in the round, including support required by carers;
>
> - design of a "care package" in agreement with users, carers and relevant agencies, to meet identified needs within the care resources available, including help from willing and able carers. Any preferred solutions which prove unavailable either because of resource constraints or because the services have not been developed will be fed back into the planning process;
>
> - implementation and monitoring of the agreed package; review of the outcomes for users and carers; any necessary revision of service provision."

The guidance also explains;

> "Care management is based on a needs led approach which has two aspects:
>
> - a progressive separation of the tasks of assessment to those of service provision in order to focus on needs, where possible having the tasks carried out by different staff;
>
> - a shift of influence from those providing to those purchasing services."

In distinguishing between care management and CPA the guidance states:

> "Where service users and carers are not provided with a single care manager, there should always be a nominated worker to act as a primary source of contact in resolving any difficulties, even if that worker changes in the course of the care management process. This equates with the arrangements for those receiving specialist psychiatric care, as set out in the care programme approach... Where complex needs are involved, this role should normally be undertaken by a care manager from the most appropriate discipline"

This difference in roles between case managers and key workers was similarly referenced in the Department's guidance on the care programme approach[1].

The existence of two different initiatives aimed at planning and managing care in the community had caused some confusion amongst professionals involved in the mental health area.

> "...given that joint working is one of the most difficult exercises everywhere, to have one requirement on one authority and a second requirement on another authority, which are almost the same but not quite, has been unhelpful and has actually confused the issue." (Health service manager)

> "I sometimes wonder if CPA is a way of evolving care management. That the ultimate aim of CPA is to make sure than the most disabled and ill people do not slip through the net. It was all basically a response to a lot of media criticism of mentally ill people on the street and CPA is a way of identifying those people who are most ill, most likely to upset the local MP or the neighbours and try to identify those needs and meet those needs. And CPA seems to ultimately filter down to care management." (Health service manager)

> "If a social worker simply does an assessment and it doesn't require care management, will they carry on delivering the service or commissioning the service or organising it and how is that different from being a care manager? -We are in the process of making sense of that." (Social services manager)

Although there was a general awareness that CPA required a health authority lead and care management was the responsibility of social services departments, there were widely varying interpretations of how CPA and care management differed - and the ways in which they interlocked.

> " It's (care management) an extension of it (CPA), it's the most ill part of it if you like. Its the furthest down the road that you can get with the new approach - the end of the road..I like to look at care management as the most specialised piece myself... there is a great big circle which is CPA and a little circle within which is care management... care management comes from the care programme approach" (Care manager)

> "There shouldn't be any difference... this is why it is almost a nonsense to have the two programmes; Because it is the same thing ie multi-agency liaison and care... I think it's fairly clear at the moment. I mean it's clear from the health side and the social services side which is which; If it is care

---

1   The Annex to circular HC/90/23 states that '... it is necessary to have effective arrangements both for monitoring that the agreed services are,indeed,provided, and for keeping in contact with the patient and drawing attention to his or her condition. This is a narrower concept than that of case management as envisaged in the White paper "caring for People" and upon which specific guidance will shortly be given to authorities.

programme they (health) are doing it. If it's care management social services are doing it, or will be doing it" (MIND)

"They (CPA, community clinical assessment, care management) are being talked about as though they are all different things but they are actually all a process being done to the same person, I feel...but it is not yet being seen as a continuum" (Health service manager)

"They have it in their mind that there is a whole group of people who are chronically disabled and in need of some sort of assessment and care management, who are separate from another group of people who tend to go in and out of hospital or who have contact with psychiatry - that's not the case, they are the same people and to have these two approaches is silly." (Consultant psychiatrist)

To a large extent, these differences of interpretation were a result of the degree to which planning for care management and planning for CPA had been linked; and the extent to which plans for care management had progressed.

In two areas, CPA planning had proceeded apart from planning for care management. In a third area, it was regarded as very important that care management and CPA be developed together. Thus they were considered by the same working group and the CPA policy document made frequent mention of care management. In the fourth area, CPA and care management were seen as almost interchangeable, in terms of ground level practice, and the policy document referred to both as such. However social services here were developing a separate care management policy.

The area that felt CPA and care management should be developed simultaneously had advanced the implementation of care management. Care managers were already being appointed and a screening process had been adopted which determined whether a patient would receive care programme approach (ie a keyworker) or whether they would receive care management. In the other three areas the care programme approach was being implemented in advance of care management.

The main dimensions on which CPA and care management were compared and contrasted concerned the target groups, the role of care managers or key workers, and the processes involved in care planning and care delivery. These are all issues that are dealt with in detail in the following sections and the overlaps or differences between the two initiatives are considered there.

2.4 Summary

- CPA was felt to embrace and formalise good practice.

- A number of potential advantages of implementing CPA were identified;

  - More systematic assessment of patients' needs

- Improvement in the quality of discharge planning

- Enhancement of inter-agency and multi-disciplinary working

- Encouragement of a more client centred approach

- Promotion of accountability for aftercare

- Identification of missing resources

- There was some resistance to the concept of CPA as;

    - Bureaucratic and overstructured

    - Impinging on clinical practice and judgement

    - A government imposed procedure

- There were also concerns that CPA would be;

    - Over inclusive ie unnecessary in some areas or for some patients

    - Unrealistic to implement without extra resources, both in terms of staff time needed to carry out the procedures and community resources required.

- The existence of two different initiatives, CPA and care management, aimed at planning and managing care in the community, had caused some confusion. The two initiatives had only been integrated in one area.

CHAPTER 3 Developing and Progressing the Implementation of CPA

The proposal to introduce the care programme approach was announced in the 1989 white paper 'Caring for People'. Its institution was planned to take place in April 1991. In the preceding September, the Department of Health issued guidance on the implementation of CPA through circular HC (90) 23, previously referenced.

This chapter considers how the four authorities developed policies and plans for CPA and some of the issues encountered in doing so. It also describes the stage that implementation had reached by the late summer of 1992 and the factors that were influencing its progress.

3.1 Policies and Plans for Introducing CPA

The formulation of CPA policies and plans took place alongside a number of other developments affecting health authorities and social service departments. Some of these, for example the implementation of the Children Act, were common to all authorities. Others, such as meeting DHA directives on discharge policy, the restructuring of mental health services and hospital applications for Trust status, were specific to individual study areas at the time. All of them, however, required the time and energy of senior staff, some of whom were key players in the implementation of CPA. This had affected both the speed of planning for CPA and the level of support lent to it.

Timescale

In three of the four areas, planning had begun following the issue of the Department's guidance on the implementation of CPA in September 1990. Although some discussion of CPA had taken place at management level prior to this, it was at this time that lead officers were identified and working groups established. In the fourth, area a working group had been formed some time before the receipt of the circular.

First drafts of CPA policy documents were formulated by October 1990 in two areas and by March 1991 in the other two authorities. In all areas, policy documents were subsequently modified through the process of consultation and piloting.

The timescale allowed for planning for CPA - generally seen as the time between the distribution of the circular in September 1990 and the implementation date, April 1st 1991 - was felt by many to be too short to complete the task in hand.

> "A circular which comes out in mid-September the year before, by the time it has been to the regions and got circulated down, most of the people who needed to see it didn't until autumn time and there were lots of other issues

going on at the same time, so that it did seem like a short time span"
(Social services manager)

Due to the short timeframe, policies had been developed more quickly than some of those involved would have liked. It was felt that insufficient time had been allowed for the lengthy process of convening working groups, consultation and planning. One result of this was that policies were translated too quickly into operational procedures. Some of the plans developed were thus unworkable or failed to address key issues. For example, at an early stage, one health services manager commented that, had the timeframe been more manageable, she would have liked to address issues such as multidisciplinary working and the role of the key worker initially, and then progress on to the procedural considerations at a later stage.

Responsibility for Planning

Approaches to planning varied both in terms of the roles of the health authorities and social services departments and the profession and seniority of those who took the lead role.

The extent of joint planning

In two areas, both the health authority and social services department were involved in the planning of CPA from its inception and joint policies were prepared. In a third area the initial policy and forms were drafted by an exclusively health authority working group and then put out to the local authorities for consultation. Once the local authorities agreed to the policy, joint working groups were set up with each to facilitate its implementation.

In the fourth area a social services department had taken the lead to prepare a CPA policy. It had done this in the absence of any action from the health authorities with which it was associated. A senior social services officer in the area felt that the health authority's inactivity stemmed from a combination of factors including staff cuts, concentration on trust status for a hospital and a recent NHS inspection. The lack of leadership by the health authority had caused some resentment within the social service department.

A second social services department in this area had not become involved until after the policy document had been written and agreed. This, according to a senior officer, was a common scenario; any joint planning tended to be carried out in this manner, which resulted in inadequate consultation about the needs of his own department's clients.

> *"Historically there has been a dearth of joint planning facilities between the health authority and the local authority and therefore, when you've got something new like this, you've virtually got to start from scratch. It's extremely difficult ... it's not as if you've got a history of good consultative working together where everybody knows who everyone is and what their*

roles are, what their expectations are - and you can press on and get a piece of work done."

Allocation of the Lead Role/s

In the three areas where the health authority had taken the appropriate lead in developing CPA, senior management had been assigned responsibility for policy and planning. In the fourth area the lead was taken, by default, by senior officers from the social services department.

Because of the level of input required, lead officers in two areas had found it necessary to delegate responsibility for the day to day development of CPA to more junior staff. In one case, a new full time position had been created with the role of educating relevant staff about CPA's aims and procedures, gathering and reporting on monitoring information to the management group and facilitating discussion of quality standards for discharge planning. This post came into being in mid 1991 and it was envisaged that the post holder would be responsible for assisting in the implementation of both CPA and care management. In the other area, the responsibility for CPA was added to an existing planning and development post. The officer here was assisted by a newly created half time post which was filled by a CPN. Their manager felt that it was very important to organise planning in this way:

> *"If you just have a working group and produce papers and push them out you will get nowhere with it"*

In the other two areas responsibility for CPA planning on a day to day basis stayed with the senior managers (assisted by members of the working groups). The additional time needed to plan, educate staff, and deal with the practical aspects of implementation created extremely heavy workloads for these managers. One of them commented at an early stage that it would have been preferable to appoint one person to look exclusively at discharge and aftercare. This more concentrated focus would have aided planning and implementation.

Forums for Planning

In all areas, a working group was established to address the issues raised by CPA. Three of these were joint committees with both health authority and social services representatives. The fourth was initially limited to health authority staff only, with joint groups being established once a draft policy had been circulated. Representatives from social services were not involved initially as it was felt important that health took the lead and *"got their own house in order"* first. Restructuring taking place in one of the SSDs here also meant that their attention was focused elsewhere.

In two of the areas the working groups used were already in existence. In one case the group had been focusing on the implementation of aftercare for patients coming under Section 117. The other group had been set up to implement care management prior to the change in timetable for this initiative.

The composition of these groups varied from area to area. However they generally included the lead managers, development officers (where relevant), consultant psychiatrists, clinical psychologists, nurse managers, senior social workers and their managers and ward managers. In one area the medical records officer was involved because of the importance assigned to centralised records in the operation of CPA. Occupational therapists were only represented on one of the working groups.

In one area consultants were not represented on the working group. There seemed to be some difference of view as to whether they had been invited. However, the consultants had felt that the issue needed to be put to the Division of Psychiatry for discussion. Further meetings of the working group were thus held without input from this group.

The FHSA was represented on the working group in just one area. At first they had played a peripheral role but had subsequently become more involved. There were plans to begin circulating information to GPs about CPA through the FHSA newsletter. In two other areas, some GPs had been involved in the planning process to a very limited extent through, for example, attendance at a joint planning meeting.

The working groups had generally been productive and had considered a wide range of issues relating to CPA and wider issues such as care management. There had, however, been some difficulties in convening groups, finding the time to attend groups and with the slow pace of progress being made to operationalise CPA. The latter problem had, in one area, been caused by many changes in group membership. In another area, progress had been impaired by the non-attendance of senior health authority staff at key meetings.

Documents Produced

Policy documents for CPA were prepared in all areas. These outlined the background to, and aims of, CPA and the response of the health authority and social services department/s. All included copies of forms to be used in the administration of CPA.

Although all of the documents were similar in structure, their focus varied. In two of the areas, for example, the approach to CPA was strongly linked with the concept of care management and the policy documents stressed the importance of compatibility between the two. A senior manager in one of these areas commented that co-operation between health and social services was enhanced by the strategy of planning CPA as a complement to care management. Another area had initially prepared a policy document based on existing Section 117 (Mental Health Act 1983) procedures. Section 117 procedure was adopted as a starting point as this was a policy already in existence and one with which people were familiar. It was hoped that this would minimise any resistance.

Early consultations

In all areas, individuals outside of the working groups were consulted at an early stage about the proposed CPA policies. This occurred in a variety of ways.

In one area, a series of half day workshops took place in April 1991. These were open to all interested health authority and social services staff and were well attended by ward managers, social workers, psychologists, administrators, managers and all of the consultants. The policy document was amended following these workshops and circulated again for comment.

In another area the draft policy document was circulated to staff at management level in both the health authority and social services department. It was then discussed within the various professional groups and feedback given to the working group. The issues raised were addressed in a subsequent version of the policy.

In a third area, the lead officers from both the health authority and social services department visited the community mental health teams to consult staff about CPA.

In the fourth area, open meetings were held in addition to the working groups. Attendance at these groups, however, had been low, with CPNs and operational managers being the main supporters. Consultation with psychiatrists took place on an individual level as well as via the Division of Psychiatry.

Representatives of the voluntary sector (MIND and NSF) were involved at the planning stage in three of the four areas. In one they were consulted through a mental health forum which was led by the social services department. In another area, a voluntary organisation formed part of the working group and in a third the policy was sent to a local agency for comment.

Piloting

In two of the four areas, procedures for CPA were piloted before being introduced across the services as a whole. In both cases, piloting took place on an acute ward and feedback had been used to modify the policies and plans. In a third area, CPA was piloted on a rehabilitation ward in the neighbouring health authority with which the study health authority shared a common policy. In the fourth area, there was no specific plan to test CPA procedures before they were introduced.

Role of Departmental and other guidance

During the planning stage for CPA, familiarity with the DoH guidance varied. Those in lead roles were generally familiar with the content of the circular while others, including members of management, consultants and other professionals had little, if any, awareness of its specific requirements.

The guidance was generally felt to leave CPA very much open to interpretation by individual authorities. This was, for the most part, welcomed, and there were few requests for more prescriptive guidance. It was felt that this would not allow local conditions to be taken into account and may thus render implementation more difficult. Some professionals however felt that there should have been greater clarification on specific issues, such as the reference group and methods of assessment. A few also argued that some lead development work on CPA would have been useful so that case studies of methods and procedures could have been provided as examples.

In one area the regional health authority issued its own guidance on CPA in February 1991. This guidance had had more impact than the Departmental circular, as the former stipulated more clearly what was required from CPA. The regional guidance was welcomed as "tightening up" the principles set out in the Department's circular. Those involved in CPA planning for the area had also found the close liaison with the RHA social service adviser very useful. In addition the RHA had organised seminars at which representatives from each district reported on their progress with CPA and discussed the issues arising. These again were welcomed.

However, guidance coming from the RHA and the Department were felt to be contradictory in certain respects. For example, the RHA sent a memo in response to the request of consultants for clarification about assessment. This memo was understood as stating that CPA only required a simple assessment system. It added that assessment did not necessarily mean that a doctor had to see a patient, but could instead be carried out using the patient's notes. It was felt that the Department's circular suggested that more complex systems and procedures should be set up.

3.2   Progress on Implementation by September 1992

As noted previously, the second stage of investigation for this research took place between May and September 1992. By this time, CPA had been implemented, to varying degrees of completeness, in three of the four authorities. In the fourth health authority there had been virtually no progress in the intervening period and the care programme approach was still not yet in operation.

The next part of the report will be looking in detail at the stage of implementation that had been reached and at judgements about how successfully it was operating. Before turning to this more detailed account, it is important to consider some of the factors that helped or hindered the general progress of the initiative. These were, in fact, numerous, but those of clearly key significance surrounded the following issues.

Relationships between health authorities and social service departments

It is a recurrent theme in any appraisal of community care initiatives that progress is best made in authorities where there are strong mechanisms between health and social service authorities for joint planning and development of services. These have to exist at both management and operational levels and need to be accompanied by equal levels of commitment to the provision of community mental health services.

The two health authorities that had most fully developed joint working at ground level for CPA had co-terminous catchment areas with their local authorities. There was therefore only one social service department to liaise with and in both there were reasonably sound structures for joint planning. In one of the two however, the social services department was considered by the health authority to be trailing in its commitment to and resourcing of community mental health services and this had led to some difficulties in progressing aspects of the care programme approach. In the other co-terminous authority where there had been highly integrated development of CPA and care management, there were also some criticisms of the level of social services resourcing of these initiatives.

In the authority that had not progressed CPA there had been a low level of involvement in joint planning at a senior level from the health authority, both on this initiative and more generally. This had been the source of some frustration to the linked social services departments, one of which had tried to take the lead on CPA.

The need for a sustained lead

There was an almost unanimous view that there had to be a 'driving force' to make the implementation of the CPA effective. This was a role that was seen to belong to the lead officers who, in the view of many, had to be people with sufficient seniority to ensure that CPA worked on a day to day basis.

> "It has got to be somebody who is authoritative enough and respected enough to deal with the other disciplines. You can't just get in a grade 2 clerk to run it because they wouldn't have the clout to make sure that people did it. That would have to be a system where people were happy to do it and they just had to pass the stuff on. So it has got to be a fairly senior person to take it on." (Consultant psychiatrist)

Another essential requirement was that the momentum behind the initiative should be sustained. It was not sufficient for CPA to be introduced and then left with the hope that it would happen. Again, it was argued that there needed to be someone with sufficient authority who would continually review its progress. This, in the view of many, required the full time attention of a senior manager.

The need for a forceful and sustained lead on CPA was well exemplified in the four authorities studied. Progress had clearly been greatest when there had been infusions of this kind from senior staff. Conversely, in the authority that had not yet implemented the CPA, there had been little apparent drive from senior management on the health side. In no authority, however, had it been possible to commit a senior officer to the work full time. It was this that led to consistent criticism of the Department for the expectation that CPA could be implemented effectively without assigning some additional resources.

Role of key professionals

Across the four authorities there were clearly very different levels of commitment to CPA among professional staff. As a group, consultants were seen to have the lowest level of enthusiasm for the initiative and this was certainly confirmed directly by some of them. In all of the authorities, some consultants were criticised for their apparent lack of interest in, or 'ownership' of CPA. This, in the view of other professionals, was affecting the pace at which CPA could be implemented.

> *"I think the problem with all my dealings with consultants is that you don't usually have a problem if you get early ownership. But with this document it was impossible to get an early ownership. It was there and if there is one thing that doctors resent its anything that is seen to impinge on their clinical freedom...."* (Health services manager)

> *"One of the faults right from the beginning was that the medical staff had little input or training. They are key personnel in terms of discharge decisions and after care but they weren't committed to CPA or the procedures involved. They gave the impression that they felt they had to do it but it was just a paper exercise, often a lot of fumbling with the paper work in a dismissive way, 'what's this form for?', or 'What do I do with this?' sort of attitude."* (CPN)

There were, however, some notable exceptions and where consultants had given some impetus to CPA its implementation had substantially progressed.

> *"Certainly Dr..... has co-operated almost begrudgingly - he has said 'Yes, ok', but he's not putting a lot of energy into making the system work and, in fact, he has been quite cynical about it, whereas Dr..... has taken it on board quite enthusiastically."* (Health services manager)

Other key professionals had had a similar impact on the success of CPA implementation. This was particularly so for people in more senior positions such as service or directorate managers, ward managers or service development officers. One reason for this was that they were able to demonstrate the importance of CPA to staff at other levels, which in turn helped to encourage the adoption of its associated procedures.

A useful example of how the input of more senior staff could help to speed the progress of CPA was found in one of the two authorities where CPA had been introduced for elderly people with mental illness. The consultant responsible for elderly services had been enthusiastic about the principles of care programming and had given high priority to its introduction. Support for the initiative was shared by the service manger, key ward managers and by the officer in charge of the CMHT for elderly people. Largely as a consequence of this, CPA had been introduced and become fully implemented in the elderly wards over a period of about six months.

Induction and training

The staff working at operational levels were generally critical of the way in which the care programme approach had been introduced to them and the training they had in CPA procedures. This was true of all three authorities where CPA had been introduced, although mechanisms for training had been changed and improved.

There were a number of different features of the induction process that received criticism. These included insufficient consultation or information prior to the introduction of CPA, forms and procedures that were continually being changed, a lack of introduction to the purpose of CPA and, in some cases, the absence of any training at all.

> "There was little training on it and it was quite noticeable when it first came in. Later on last year, when we were supposed to be doing it officially, the junior doctors on our ward did not know what the meetings were...you went out and you found out what you were supposed to be doing and they were all really angry... If you are in the right place at the right time you hear about it. Its all hearsay. But if you are not in the right place at the right time you have had it basically." (Occupational therapist)

> "They were far behind developing CPA in .....(authority) and then it was imposed. It was going to happen on ....(start date). This was 3 days previous and nobody (on the wards) knew anything about it." (Ward manager)

An important outcome of adequate consultation, induction and training was that CPA and its procedures became accepted and integrated by the professionals who had to administer them. Without commitment of this kind, systems for implementing CPA could easily be forgotten or ignored under the pressures of other work. This had clearly slowed up the introduction of CPA in certain parts of the service in all the three authorities currently operating CPA. Conversely, where there had been effective training and induction programmes, the implementation of CPA had progressed.

Review and progress chasing

There was a consistent view among all professionals that CPA procedures needed continuing review and monitoring to aid their introduction. Without it, implementation was likely to be patchy or non-existent. Moreover, it was argued that progress of the system had to happen at both management and operational levels.

> *"It isn't happening as widely as it should... it will need pressure... if it doesn't get sufficient of a hold then it won't spread - everyone will think 'Well, nobody else is doing it, why should we?'... I think people need to go out and say 'This is what ought to be done' and encourage people to do it through workshops with the nurses, getting them to do their bit, meeting with the medics and saying, 'Right, these are the final forms', rather than just sending them a cold letter. I think it needs face to face contact"* (Consultant psychiatrist)

> *"It's like anything - if you leave it for long enough it will probably fall apart. Depends on the person running the ward to make sure these things happen but if you get new people coming in and they are not sure what to do, it might not get done and it will gradually fall apart... We need some further small workshops to say what we are doing, how we are doing it, whether it is working or not, where we can get some feedback on all of this form filling we have done..."* (Ward manager, acute)

This call for some monitoring and feedback on how the system was working was a recurrent one. The importance of this is further discussed in Chapter 8.

3.3 Summary

- The Department of Health's circular on CPA was issued in September 1990 and implementation was expected to take place by April 1991. There was some feeling that this timetable was too short, resulting in policies which failed to address some of the key issues.

- Implementation was going on in the context of many other developments, both national and local, in health and social services management. CPA had had to compete with these for development time.

- In two areas planning took place jointly, with both the health authority and social services involved from the outset. In a third the health authority began the process and then included social services. In the fourth area, social services took the lead.

- Overall responsibility for implementing CPA was taken by senior staff. In two areas, however, the day to day implementation was delegated to development officers because of the amount of input needed. This was widely acknowledged to be a desirable strategy.

- Joint working groups had been established to develop CPA policy. These covered a wide range of issues and were generally felt to be productive. Staff at various levels in the health authorities and social services departments were involved and, to a lesser extent, representatives of voluntary agencies, users and FHSAs/GPs.

- Policy documents were prepared in all areas and consultation with health, social services and other staff took place. In two areas the CPA policy was piloted on an acute ward before full implementation.

- Departmental guidance was felt to leave wide scope for interpretation. For the most part this was welcomed and the need to tailor plans to fit local circumstances was highlighted. More prescriptive guidance from the Department was not required. However, case studies and examples of good practice, as could have been generated by some lead development work, would have been useful.

- CPA had been implemented, to varying degrees of completeness, in three of the four health authorities. A number of factors had had an influence on the progress of implementation;

  - The relationship between the health authority and social services department/s, in particular the strength of joint planning.

  - The need for a sustained lead or driving force having the authority to further the implementation.

  - The level of commitment to, and ownership of, CPA, particularly amongst groups such as consultants and unit or service managers who had the potential to engender enthusiasm amongst ward and community staff.

  - The level of induction and training; There was some criticism of the lack of information provided on the principles and practice of CPA. This, in some cases, had contributed to a lack of commitment.

  - There was a need for the progress of CPA to be reviewed and followed up regularly to prevent patchy implementation and to provide feedback to staff and management.

PART II

OPERATING THE CARE PROGRAMME APPROACH

CHAPTER 4 The Targeting of CPA

All of the authorities studied recognised that CPA should cover all in-patients considered for discharge and all new patients accepted by the specialist psychiatric services after 1st April 1991, as specified by the circular. Each, however, had to consider how this statement should be interpreted in view of the structure and resources of their service.

In each area the policy document relating to CPA set out which patients would have their needs for aftercare assessed. Although selection and inclusion criteria varied slightly from authority to authority there were some key points common to all CPA plans.

4.1 Policies on Inclusion of Individual Patients in CPA

Although the Department of Health circular stated that CPA should apply to "all in-patients considered for discharge, and all new patients accepted by the specialist psychiatric services", there was some misunderstanding about what constituted CPA and, therefore, who was included in it. CPA was often believed to require a complex care plan in which two or more professions were involved. Patients who were assessed as needing simpler aftercare, for example an out-patients appointment and/or visits from a CPN only, could thus be seen as being outside CPA.

The policy documents, in each area, indicated that *all* in-patients were to have their community care needs assessed within CPA procedures[1]. Thus, in theory, no patient should leave hospital without a decision being made about the level and nature of aftercare required, a decision which would ideally be made by a multi-disciplinary team. However, if patients were not considered to be "vulnerable" or to have sufficiently complex needs to warrant inclusion in CPA, this decision, and the subsequent arrangements made for aftercare (for example, an out-patients appointment) may not be recorded. This meant that the information did not become part of a central CPA record and could not be used to ensure systematic reviewing of the care plans or to assist management in future planning.

In three of the authorities there was a formal provision for the multi-disciplinary team to decide that a patient was not "vulnerable" or did not have "enduring mental health problems". In this case a multi-disciplinary aftercare plan was not considered necessary and patients concerned were followed up by one single professional (for example a CPN, psychologist, a psychiatrist at out-patients and/or their GP). In

---

1 Some in-patients, however, remained in hospital as it was known that suitable facilities, usually accommodation, were not available for them at that time in the community. Their needs in relation to living in the community were not, however, fully assessed until the presence of suitable accommodation made leaving hospital an option.

two areas it was intended that this decision would be recorded on the CPA paperwork and provision had been made on the appropriate forms to do so. The aftercare arrangements themselves, however, may not be recorded, and keyworkers and review dates may not be arranged.

In the fourth area there was no formal provision for patients to be screened out of the CPA process at this stage and everyone discharged from hospital was expected to have a written care plan[1]. There was evidence, however, that some informal screening out took place at ward level.

Strategies for determining whether a formal aftercare plan was needed for any given patient varied. For example, in one area a nine point check list was administered by ward staff. This focused on the patient's history of care, including number of admissions to hospital and length of stay, use of day hospital or day centre, length of contact with psychiatric services, use of major tranquilisers, use of sheltered accommodation and ability to carry out functions of daily living. Patients having a certain score against such criteria were to be regarded as having "enduring mental health problems". However this was intended to be used as a guideline only and there was room for discretion as the multi-disciplinary team had the final say.

In another area, there was no formal strategy of this type but ward staff spoke of taking into account similar factors in deciding whether a patient was "vulnerable" and in need of an aftercare plan. The importance of considering the nature of the illness, particularly whether it was chronic or a single acute episode unlikely to be repeated, was also pointed out here. In a third area, a care plan was to be drawn up when input from more than one agency was assessed to be needed.

4.2 The Stage of Implementation of CPA across Mental Health Services

The extent to which CPA had been implemented at the time of the research varied between the study areas and between different parts of the service within each authority. In all areas implementation was taking place in phases in order to make it more manageable. In-patient services were targeted at first, and once CPA was well established, people already living in the community and in touch with the mental health services would be included. Implementation was not yet fully complete in any of the study areas. The reasons for this were outlined in detail in Chapter 3.

In-patients

In one area there had been no implementation of the CPA policy. In the other three it had been implemented for in-patients in the acute, rehabilitation

---

1   There had initially been a policy of including only sectioned and "vulnerable" patients in CPA discharge planning but this had been extended to include all patients, as originally planned, in April 1992.

and long stay facilities. In two areas elderly in-patients were also included[1]. Some specialist in-patient services were included (eg a mother and baby unit). However there was still some question as to whether the child and adolescent services should practice CPA.

Although CPA had been officially implemented for all in-patients discharged from hospital, several instances were described where assessment and discharge planning were not happening. Thus the following of CPA policy was, in some cases, a "hit and miss affair". Three main factors influenced the extent to which CPA was being implemented for the intended clients; pressure of work, staff awareness of CPA procedures, and the motivation of staff to implement the new system. The extent to which CPA paperwork had been completed in one area, for example, was monitored as part of the nursing audit and it had been found that implementation varied between wards. This was attributed to a combination of the relative busyness of the wards and differences from ward to ward in staff awareness of and attitudes towards CPA.

- Pressure of work

  Decisions as to who would receive assessment under CPA could be related to the resources available, either in the hospital or in the community, rather than the needs of patients. On the in-patient side, for example, ward staff described how pressure of work made it difficult to find the time to assess the aftercare needs of all patients. People staying in hospital for a short time only (see Section 4.3) and longer stay patients in busy acute wards were two groups specifically highlighted as likely to be missed out because of this.

  A shortage of resources in the community was also felt likely to limit the numbers who could receive planned aftercare. Many community staff from both the health authorities and social services reported caseloads already stretched to the limit and waiting lists. Given the central part played in CPA by these staff, this could also limit its scope.

- Staff awareness of CPA procedure

  Some professionals, including consultants and ward staff, were not aware of how to use the CPA forms and paperwork may not have been completed or may have been left to those who were believed to be more au fait with the procedures.

- Staff motivation to implement CPA procedures

  In some cases there was a reluctance by staff to apply CPA procedures. This might be because they did not feel that they were necessary, for example where the patient was not considered to have sufficiently complex needs (see Section 4.2). Low motivation could also arise from a lack of training, so that staff were not aware of the purpose of CPA and/or the related procedures (see Chapter 3).

---

1   In the third area elderly services were under different management and CPA had not yet been implemented

Some of the implications of such variations in practice were reported to be;

- Little or no implementation of CPA procedures where, for example, a consultant was lacking in knowledge of what was expected

- Inconsistency of communication about CPA, for example, in convening multi-disciplinary meetings

- Marked differences between wards and/or individual members of staff in the numbers of people referred on to care management

Users of mental health services living in the community

All the authorities intended to extend CPA to those already living in the community. Thus people using the mental health services through out-patients, CMHTs, day hospitals and centres or their GP were eventually to be involved. To date, the implementation within these parts of the service varied.

- Community Mental Health Teams

  One CMHT for the elderly was applying CPA to all referrals, whether or not they were in-patients. The CMHTs in another area had been using multi-disciplinary assessments for some time but were not using the procedures defined in the CPA policy.

- Day hospital patients

  These were included in CPA in two areas.

- Out-patients

  In one area CPA had been extended to include out-patients and there was a suggestion that this should happen in another. There was some resistance to this amongst consultants, however, who felt that it was quite unnecessary. A large proportion of out-patients referred directly by GPs were thought unlikely to be in need of a care plan. The requirement to fill in paperwork to say that they were the only professional involved was not regarded as a good use of consultants' time.

- Patients not referred to a consultant psychiatrist

  There had been some debate as to whether out-patient cases referred directly by GPs to the CPN or psychology services, for example, should be included in CPA. There was a widespread belief that if a client was not in need of a consultant psychiatrist it was unlikely that their needs for aftercare were sufficiently complex to warrant assessment under CPA. Such patients tended to have one-off episodes of illness, perhaps in response to a personal crisis, or were people already functioning reasonably well in the community. These groups were only formally excluded from CPA in one authority although in the others they were unlikely to be included for the above reasons.

4.3 Groups for whom CPA Implementation was Difficult

There were some groups of in-patients for whom it was difficult to ensure that assessment of aftercare needs under CPA took place. These included those discharging themselves against medical advice, those refusing aftercare, those spending a very short time in hospital and those with no fixed abode. Arrangements for dealing with these situations were often not formalised and varied both within and between authorities.

Patients not wanting aftercare

Some patients did not wish to receive any aftercare. This was an issue often mentioned in connection with people who discharged themselves, but could also apply to those whose discharge was planned. Such situations were difficult to deal with. The consensus concerning this group was that little could be done and, in some cases, it was inevitable that they would lose touch with the mental health services. In one area, the user's agreement to be included in CPA was part of the policy.

Patients discharging themselves

Where patients discharged themselves early against medical advice but were not refusing further care, attempts were often made by hospital staff to arrange some form of aftercare. For example, this could include informing the GP, and any other agencies known to be involved, that the person is discharged, or arranging a follow-up visit from a CPN if this was felt necessary.

The above two groups were a source of concern, especially as it was suspected that vulnerable patients with long term needs may leave hospital prematurely and opt out of an aftercare plan due to the nature of their illness and their lack of insight into it. People felt to be particularly at risk here were young schizophrenics and those with behavioural or personality disorders.

Short stay patients

There were a number of differing views about the logistics of providing multi-disciplinary assessment and discharge planning for those who came into hospital for a few days only. Although short stay patients were not officially excluded from CPA in any of the areas, it was likely to be difficult to arrange this prior to discharge due to time constraints.

Some professionals were of the opinion that CPA was not necessary for short term patients as, by definition, they were unlikely to have continuing care needs. For example they may have been admitted for assessment and found to have a personality disorder or a crisis related condition rather than a long term mental illness.

Where follow-up care was felt to be needed, however, the issue could be addressed by inviting the person back to the ward in the first few weeks following discharge to discuss their progress or by following up with a visit from community staff.

There was some feeling that it was not possible to apply CPA to very short stay patients, particularly those leaving quickly following a tribunal decision or those not already known to the services. A lack of both resources to follow up such cases and time available to assess their needs while in-patients were given as reasons for this.

Homeless people/people living in temporary accommodation/people from outside the area

"*Slipping through the net*" was often associated with homeless or transient people living in inner-city areas. Staff from the two authorities not covering inner-city areas felt that this was not an issue for their areas as very few of their patients lived in these circumstances.

In one health authority covering an inner city area, however, people with no fixed abode or living in temporary bed and breakfast accommodation were acknowledged to be difficult to keep in touch with. For example, out-patients appointments were often not kept and the patients concerned may not be seen again following discharge until a future emergency prompted hospitalisation.

The situation was compounded for patients who were not permanently resident in the area or who circulated from authority to authority. In this case it was sometimes difficult to establish which health or local authority had responsibility for their care in the community. A shortage of social work resources could make it difficult for the necessary "detective work" to be carried out in establishing aftercare services available, other than in cases where there was a statutory requirement to do so. Ward staff and consultants did, however, take on some of this role themselves, although aftercare planning and follow-up under these circumstances was difficult.

CPA, then, has been implemented for in-patients and there are intentions to extend this further to those already living in the community. However, it is clear that where implementation has taken place, not every patient in contact with the service receives CPA. There are also certain groups of service users who are likely to fall outside the CPA procedures unless special arrangements are made to ensure their inclusion.

4.4 Summary

-    In the three areas where CPA had been implemented, acute, rehabilitation and long stay patients were included. In some cases in-patient EMI services were also covered as well as some specialist units eg mother and baby.

- Implementation for people already in the community was following behind that for in-patients. Some implementation had taken place in CMHTs, out-patients, day hospitals and there were intentions to extend this further.

- *All* in-patients were to have their needs for aftercare assessed in a multi-disciplinary setting. In three areas this initial assessment was to be used to screen out those who are not considered to need a formal care plan, keyworker, review etc. There was some misunderstanding as to what constituted CPA and who, therefore, should be included in it. CPA was often believed to require a complex care plan. Those needing just and out-patients appointment, for example, were sometimes regarded as being outside CPA's remit.

- Time constraints for both ward and community staff were a major reason why the multi-disciplinary assessment and planning of aftercare may not be possible in some cases.

- Levels of motivation and awareness amongst staff in relation to CPA could also influence how consistently it was implemented.

- Patients discharging themselves, refusing aftercare, in hospital for a short stay or having no fixed abode could be difficult to include in CPA.

- People with one-off episodes of illness, perhaps crisis related, were a group commonly felt not to need CPA.

CHAPTER 5   Assessment and Discharge Planning

In each area where CPA had been introduced, procedures had been
established for assessing patients' needs in the community and
formulating a plan of care to meet these. A multi-disciplinary
discussion in which a keyworker was appointed and decisions made
about aftercare formed the basis of assessment and discharge planning.
However, practice varied in details such as the forum used for planning,
the nature of the assessments, documentation of procedures and
responsibility for co-ordination and communication. In addition, the
identification of keyworkers and the staff resources needed to complete
this part of CPA raised a number of issues for both managers and
ground level staff. This chapter describes how assessment and
discharge planning was carried out and the factors affecting plans
made.

5.1   *The Nature of Assessments*

In theory the assessment of needs for aftercare and the formulation of a plan
to meet these needs were two separate elements of CPA. In two areas
this was reflected in the policy. In one health authority, two separate
meetings were required; the first soon after a patient was admitted, to
assess their needs and appoint a keyworker; and the second prior to
discharge, to finalise the care plan. In reality, however, it was said that
the former meeting often did not take place and both the individual's
needs and their care plan were discussed at one pre-discharge meeting.
In the second area assessment took place using a formalised schedule
administered by ward nurses. The results were then discussed at a
multi-disciplinary meeting where the care plan was formulated.

Many considered it preferable to begin the assessment and planning process
as soon as patients were admitted, in order to prepare for discharge.

> *"The responsibility of the keyworker is to ensure, long before the last
> meeting is convened, that they have a very good idea of what is needed. The
> home work, the ground work, the spade work should have been done. In that
> meeting you are putting the final touches or reassessing and reappraising
> the amount of time which needs to go in - we can't provide 4 days care,
> we'll provide 3 days care or whatever, but we should be aware by that time
> of what is needed. Its no good leaving it all until that time, otherwise you
> will have another three months in hospital"* (Ward manager)

It was also recognised, however, that assessments made when the patient was
first in hospital may change as their illness moves through different
stages. In one area the forms had been modified to allow for more than
one assessment during the hospital stay.

In general the final consensus on a patient's needs in the community was
established in a multi-disciplinary meeting held prior to discharge, with
the decision based on discussion of individual assessments made by the
disciplines present. There were formalised assessment schedules in one

area, as described above, and another two areas planned to move in this direction.

In the area where formalised assessment was already in place three schedules were used. The first focused primarily on the history of care received in relation to the illness and was used to screen out patients who were not perceived to have "enduring mental health problems" (see Chapter 4). Patients passing through the first assessment stage then had the extent of their continuing care needs evaluated using a further more detailed schedule. This concentrated on the patient's situation in relation to areas such as the activities of living (eg maintaining a safe environment, communications, nutrition etc), independent living (eg finance, cooking, shopping) and accommodation.

Once this assessment had been completed, conclusions were drawn about the support and care needs anticipated following discharge, the support and social care already in place and other identified areas of care and support that were needed. A scoring system attached to this assessment schedule also helped to determine whether the patient was in need of care management. If this was required the case was referred to a care manager who then carried out a more detailed assessment. There was some dissatisfaction with this system amongst some staff who felt that the scores arrived at in the assessment schedules could conflict with clinical judgement. Discussions around these schedules were on-going.

In another area, there were plans to develop a "common dependency assessment", whereby one set of assessment criteria could be used by a wide range of professionals from both health and social services.

5.2 Forum/Meetings

The multi-disciplinary discussions required by CPA took place largely as part of existing ward rounds. There were, however, some exceptions to this. For example, one consultant had arranged to meet with CPNs and social workers on a regular basis to discuss their cases, including those to be discharged in the near future. In another area the majority of pre-discharge meetings took place as part of the ward round, except where the case was particularly complex, with many different parties involved, when a separate meeting would be convened. A unit for long stay patients and an elderly care ward both held separate co-ordination meetings, apart from the ward round, where aftercare could be discussed in more detail.

There was some feeling that ward rounds were not the most appropriate forum for assessment and planning. A number of reasons were given for this;

-       They could be rushed.

        "(Ward rounds) don't enhance our contribution very much. Particularly where meetings are very rushed and there is always that feeling of processing. And we are trying to put a social perspective on the client's

circumstances, for example, about how medication fits into their life and how they are going to be supported into thinking that medication is a good thing. Ward rounds tend just to talk about what the medication is and who is doing it. There is not always time to take in the social perspective."
(Social worker)

- The numbers of people present and time limitations could make it difficult to discuss the finer details of aftercare and there may be people attending who are not directly involved.

- Ward rounds were often used as teaching sessions for medical students and planning of aftercare took second place to this.

- Ward rounds were often dominated by a consultant and focused on medical issues. It could be difficult for non-health authority staff to feel comfortable in such a setting.

- Patients could be daunted by the number of professionals and may have difficulty expressing their opinions (see Chapter 7).

Some felt that separate meetings should be convened but the logistics of this, and the importance given to ward rounds as the main forum for discussing patients, stood in the way.

5.3 *Formulation of Care Plans*

There was no formal standard governing what was or was not an adequate or minimum care plan in any of the areas. The extent to which the plans formulated were needs led could be influenced by a number of factors.

The level of resources in the community

"We are still constrained by the gap between assessed need and the facilities available to meet those needs. Of course, unmet need is not necessarily a resource issue, sometimes the client doesn't want to have a particular need met in a particular way or doesn't see it as a need. But a major area of unmet need is a resource issue. And it's, strangely enough, on the rehab side, not a resource issue in terms of health professionals, if you like, although we would obviously like more of that, but of what I would call welfare issues; reasonable accommodation, reasonable finance, reasonable freedom from exploitation and that means accommodation in a place where neighbours are accepting of that sort of thing and helpful, and those are issues we have difficulty with". (Consultant, rehabilitation)

The availability of suitable housing was usually highlighted as an important starting point for minimum care, as it was often in short supply. It was generally agreed that people should not be discharged without appropriate housing to accommodate them.

"They (hospital) are quite sympathetic when it comes to discharge. Obviously they don't want to throw you out into the wilderness. I mean, if they think you need to come to the day hospital then you'll get referred to

the day hospital. If you're homeless they wouldn't throw you out unless you had a home or were in a hostel or hotel or whatever" (Ex-patient, lost job and became homeless due to illness).

Often people with mental illness needed more than a room and a meal. For example, a representative of a voluntary organisation providing temporary accommodation described how, in some cases, their behaviour proved too disruptive or demanding of staff time to make bed and breakfast or general purpose hostels an option. Many professionals highlighted the need for specialist accommodation, in particular;

-   Staffed hostels/sheltered housing

-   Adult fostering

-   Emergency/half way accommodation specifically for people with mental illness

It was sometimes necessary to keep people in hospital while waiting for a place in a hostel, for example, to become available.

Where keeping patients in hospital for longer was not an option, however, they sometimes had to be discharged to accommodation which was felt to be less suitable.

> *"Sometimes you have to compromise because you cant get everything that you wanted in the way of support and in what the patient needs. Say you want a particular type of hostel and it is full, you have to take the next best"* (Ward manager, acute)

> *"In rehab we try and get them the most suitable accommodation but you can't do it sometimes and they go out to the Salvation Army and then get passed around all the other places that there might be but are just not suitable for them. And we know that we are sending somebody out there to live somewhere that is not suitable"* (Occupational therapist, rehabilitation)

This could lead to the people concerned coming back into hospital for the supported environment that they needed.

> *"I know some people with mental illness who have been around for years and occasionally sleep on the streets or travel around for a variety of reasons, be it their mental health or just their lifestyle. They've got themselves a reputation around the city years ago so that no-one will take them so even when they come back to us there is little that we can do. They continually go through the cyclical issue of relapse, hospitalisation, relatively settled accommodation, for example, Salvation Army, relapse, street, hospitalisation"* (Voluntary agency)

In some cases patients remained in hospital for longer than necessary because they or their relatives could not afford private sector sheltered accommodation. Thus it was necessary for them to wait until a social services run place could become available.

In addition to accommodation there were a number of areas where resources were lacking. These included;

- Health services;

    Day hospitals
    Day centres
    Sufficient transport to get patients to the above facilities
    CPN services
    Occupational therapy services in the community

- Social services

    Day centres
    Community based social workers

Some also identified a need for more care assistants to take over from qualified staff such tasks as taking clients shopping or to out-patients.

A known lack of community resources could be frustrating for ward staff who were taking the time to complete CPA paperwork without the satisfaction of knowing that there were community resources to back this up. In addition, services were sometimes offered to patients by consultants who were unaware of the resource implications in the community. For example, they may promise carers respite care for the patient when it is unlikely that this will be available. If community staff were not present at ward rounds it could be difficult for hospital staff to know what services were available.

Consideration of the full range of options available

Professionals were sometimes reported to be unwilling to consider the full range of options. This could either be due to tradition (for example seeing ward rounds as focusing on medical issues rather than social ones), or a lack of awareness of services available. In one area a checklist of services had been compiled for use in planning. This was beginning to have the effect of encouraging consultants to consider more than just an out-patients appointment as an aftercare plan.

Lack of time in acute ward rounds for discussion of aftercare

Ward rounds in acute wards were often very busy, with many patients to be discussed. The focus was also likely to be on medical issues rather than the practicalities of living in the community. Thus sometimes little time was devoted to aftercare planning (see Chapter 7).

Involving community staff in the planning at too late a stage

Sometimes community staff were not involved until just prior to the patient being discharged or even afterwards. This did not allow sufficient time for them to make a contribution to care planning or to put the necessary community resources into place.

Disagreements about who should provide care

Sometimes there were disagreements as to who should provide the care required. For example, one consultant described a case where he felt that CPN involvement was needed but the CPN disagreed. In another area a CPN believed that social work input was necessary, but this was not forthcoming.

5.4   Effect of CPA on Discharge Decisions

One of the principles of CPA is to allow people to continue with, or be admitted to, in-patient care until a minimum programme of care in the community can be arranged.

CPA was not commonly believed to have affected discharge decisions because adequate aftercare could not be provided. Discharge depended much more crucially on the level of demand for hospital beds. In the authorities where there was pressure on bed space, there was often no choice other than to discharge people, even if care plans were not entirely adequate. One health service manager in such an authority felt particularly strongly about the unrealistic demands made by this aspect of CPA;

> *"Its impossible, its just nonsense, absolute nonsense... its lunatic. I mean, if that were done seriously then there would be a very substantial increase in the number of beds required. Who will pay for them?... I mean, the District Health Authority couldn't pay for them, and we haven't got the spare money -completely impossible. In reality we don't discharge people simply onto the street, but if we were to wait until there were adequate arrangements in relation to housing, for example, there isn't any way we could actually live with that. We would have to have an awful lot more beds"*

A consultant in the same area explained that people were not discharged where circumstances would be detrimental to their welfare and that some patients were kept in hospital as resources outside were inadequate. This had to be balanced, however, with pressure on beds from suicidal patients.

In one area it was said that "lip service" was paid to this requirement of CPA

> *"Its a case of we need the bed, this person is going, we don't really care where they are going, they will probably be back in six months or less, but we will cross that bridge when we come to it"* (CPN)

Where there was less pressure on bed space, however, patients were already remaining in hospital until suitable community care provision could be found. It was recognised, however, that keeping patients in hospital longer than clinically necessary was not desirable. From the patient's point of view it could be more difficult to readjust to life in the community after long periods in hospital. Also the patient may be anxious to leave and may discharge themselves despite a shortage of community resources. From the hospital's point of view, keeping people as in-patients was costly.

Patients did sometimes remain in hospital longer than necessary while waiting for discharge planning meetings to be convened or postponed to accommodate a key professional.

5.5 *Information Recorded*

A number of documents had been put into use to record and facilitate the communication of information related to CPA. The information recorded was similar in each area and commonly included;

- The identity and contact details of the keyworker.

- The names of people present at the meeting or involved in the plan.

- Details of plans made (either in summary form or setting out separately what each profession proposes to contribute).

- The date of this and the next review meeting.

- Any resources required but not available.

- The consent or wishes of the patient and carer.

Individual areas had implemented a number of additional forms, for example;

- A number of standard letters to be sent by the ward manager to notify relevant parties of the patient's admission and entitlement to aftercare, date of probable discharge and discharge review meeting.

- A checklist of existing services in the community, with columns for recording whether these are required and, if so, whether they have been contacted.

- Schedules for recording formal assessment (see Section 5.1)

- A form for registering the patient on a central CPA record.

Forms for recording the outcome of subsequent reviews were also in use.

Copies of the completed paperwork were to be distributed to a number of points. Usually this included those involved with the care plan, although not necessarily the patient (see Chapter 7), as well as the medical records office, patient services manager and general practitioner. Some professions, however, reported that they did not receive copies of the paperwork.

There was some debate amongst professionals as to whether distributing such information was helpful. Some found it an advantage to know the name of the keyworker and to have a written outline of the plans made. Others, however, were already well aware of such details and found the information recorded too brief or incomplete to be of any real use.

The amount of paperwork, which could involve several pages, was a source of concern amongst ward staff and consultants and, in one area, there were proposals to shorten the format. Staff using the paperwork on a day to day basis sometimes found it difficult to see its purpose.

> *"If it was one piece of paper it would be brilliant but there is one part, predischarge, and that's 4 pages long.....If only a CPN attends it makes everything else look ridiculous. It's a lot of paperwork for nothing... I still have to make sure the patient has signed it or the psychologist dealing with the patient has signed it and the CPN has signed it. And then you have to photocopy it all to send to the relevant people who have agreed to do these things for the patient. So it could be either one photocopy or 10"* (Ward staff, acute)

> *"Come the 1st of April (when CPA implemented) there was a deluge of paperwork, snowed under with paperwork and it was a bit of a farce to be perfectly honest. It slowed momentum, it felt like it was losing focus and not of any practical use whatsoever, because the ones that really should have needed help were tending to be just pulled along by or subsumed by those who perhaps didn't patently need help"* (Social worker)

Those in receipt of copies of the paperwork, GPs for example, could find the number of forms cumbersome to store.

Responsibility for ensuring that CPA paperwork was completed and relevant people invited to meetings and/or informed of their outcome fell largely to the ward staff and sometimes to consultants or other doctors. However, the keyworker was expected to take on this role in one area and, in another, each profession filled out their piece of the form.

CPA paperwork placed a considerable demand on staff time, which was especially noticeable in busy acute wards. Where clerical support was in short supply, nurses had to take on CPA paperwork as part of their workload.

> *"I have two hours of clerical support per day only to file and there are six consultants....therefore the nursing staff have the responsibility to make sure that the paperwork's filled in and something has to go....My manpower resource has not altered or increased to meet that need"* (Ward manager)

This took time away from patient care and meant that either the patients missed out on nursing time or the nurses did extra work to avoid this, for example by working through their breaks.

In addition to filling in the forms, tasks such as following up other professionals to get them to complete or sign where relevant, photocopying, distributing forms and convening meetings also used up valuable time.

Ward clerks were employed in one area to complete the paperwork, establish who should be involved from the community and invite them to the appropriate meetings. There was considerable praise for this arrangement amongst professionals here who felt that CPA would be very difficult to operate without this level of clerical support. It was pointed out, however, that ward clerks did not necessarily have the expertise to know which professionals should be involved with a patient and therefore who to invite to meetings. Input from other staff was thus needed here.

In another area, however, a high staff turnover had initially made it difficult to ensure that paperwork was completed as there was insufficient continuity of staff who were aware of the procedure. A more stable core of staff had now resolved this situation. A consultant in the third health authority, however, had initially filled in the appropriate paperwork but had subsequently given this up, finding that he did not have time to continue with it.

5.6 *Identification of Keyworker*

Appointing a Keyworker

A keyworker to follow the case through into the community was usually appointed at a multi-disciplinary meeting while the patient was still in hospital. Sometimes, however, this was not possible, for example, where such a meeting did not take place or where the profession considered most appropriate to act as keyworker was not represented at the meeting. If this happened, a delay could occur while the case was referred to the CPN, social work or other services and a keyworker subsequently appointed.

> *"The community has to tell you who the keyworker is going to be and more often than not nobody comes to the meeting because there aren't the staff to come to the meeting. Everybody is angry with everybody.... Sometimes we have had a meeting and nobody has come from the community so we have got to wait until the next week so that people are staying in hospital longer"*
> (Occupational therapist, acute ward)

It was intended that the identification of the keyworker be based on a multi-disciplinary discussion and related to the patients' needs. This, however, was not always the case. For example;

- Selection could be much less formal, for example passing someone in the corridor and asking them to take on this role.

- The keyworker appointed was sometimes not present at the meeting and may not have had the opportunity to give their agreement or may have found out later that they had been appointed.

- Appointment of a keyworker could be based on the community staff present at the meeting. For example, in one area CPNs were more likely to attend meetings than social workers and were thus more likely to be appointed as keyworkers.

Very few instances were reported of cases where it had not been possible to identify a keyworker. This could, however, happen when the input of the various professions was more or less equal or where there was reluctance on the part of some professions to get involved in keyworking. Where it was not possible to appoint the keyworker felt to be the most appropriate, a substitute would be found.

A number of professionals stressed the importance of being able to change the keyworker in accordance with the changing needs of the client, for example at a review meeting.

Profession of Keyworker

Keyworkers tended to be the person who would have the most contact with the patient, usually a CPN or social worker. Where a professional had been working with the patient for some time it was often appropriate for that person to take on or continue the keyworker role.

The allocation of the keyworker also depended on the needs of the patient. In general, where housing or financial needs predominated, a social worker would take on the role, while if drug treatment or medical monitoring was the main element of care needed it could be a CPN.

In all three areas where CPA had been implemented there was some feeling that CPNs were being singled out to take on the keyworker role rather than social workers, although this was not a formal policy. This was attributed to a variety of factors including a lack of social worker resources, for example, due to attention being focussed on other issues, and a lack of understanding of CPA requirements on the part of social workers.

> "Since this care programme has been in place, I can guarantee that whenever I go up to the ward for a discharge meeting there is no discussion of who is going to be the keyworker. I can tell you before I go in the room that I have already been placed as keyworker...I may not even know the patient. You walk in and sit down and listen to what has gone on and the consultant will then say. 'Well, who shall we have as a keyworker?' And...before you can catch your breath, the social worker will say 'I think the CPN should be' and if you say 'Well, why is that? because I think you

have got more input with this client' (they say) 'Well, due to staff shortages and cutbacks, we can't provide this sort of service'" (CPN)

Conversely, in one area some believed that CPA was beginning to challenge the traditional assumption that a CPN would always take on the case. It was causing people instead to consider who was the most appropriate. Here CPA had also instigated the appointment of the keyworker prior to discharge which had not happened previously.

A consultant or other doctor might be the keyworker if they were seeing the patient frequently at out-patients and other professionals had no need to be involved. Less frequently day hospital workers, health visitors, care assistants and staff of residential facilities took on the keyworker role. In one area day hospital workers were not yet involved as keyworkers although their manager was keen for this to happen and was trying to see that they were invited to the appropriate meetings. The day hospital in another area had its own keyworker system but here the keyworkers were not expected to take on a co-ordinating role in relation to the total care package.

In one area a ward manager sometimes acted as keyworker;

> *"Sometimes we come across difficulties in identifying somebody to be the community keyworker. Usually if there is a community nurse involved then we nominate the community nurse. If there is no community nurse but a social worker then we will nominate a social worker. But sometimes the person doesn't need or want either of those two services and a lot of the time I tell them to keep in contact with myself so I am myself the keyworker, although I am not in the community"* (Ward manager, acute)

The feasibility of voluntary agencies and GPs taking on the keyworker role had not been fully addressed and they were, as yet, not generally involved in this capacity. Similarly carers were not commonly taking on the keyworker role. A representative of a voluntary agency working with carers felt that this would not be possible in any case;

> *"I can't see that working because the carer is too much involved with the patient and doesn't have any power base. There is no way that the keyworker being Mrs Jones whose son John is ill - there is no way in which Mrs Jones can cause the services to jump to it. She can put in a request but she could do that anyway"*

Although there did not seem to be a formal policy concerning this, keyworkers were generally expected to come from the statutory agencies. One reason for this was that they needed to have the necessary authority to call meetings and co-ordinate the input of several parties in the care plan.

5.7 Summary

- Procedures had been established in each area for assessing and formulating a plan of care. The basis of planning was a multi-disciplinary discussion where the keyworker was appointed and decisions made concerning aftercare.

- In theory assessment and discharge planning were separate parts of CPA. In one area there were two distinct meetings; one for assessment and one for discharge planning. However, the former did not always take place. Formalised assessment schedules were in use in another area, although in all the final consensus was usually reached in the multi-disciplinary meeting.

- Multi-disciplinary meetings took place largely in ward rounds. These were not considered to be the ideal forum for discharge planning because:

  - They could be rushed

  - There were often many people there so that it was not possible to discuss details

  - They could be dominated by medical staff, focused on medical issues and used as teaching sessions

  - Patients could be daunted by the number of professionals present.

  There was some feeling that separate meetings should be convened, although this was likely to be difficult in practice.

- No formal standard setting out minimum requirements for care plans had been established. However suitable accommodation was often highlighted as an important indicator, being in short supply.

- The extent to which plans were needs led depended on;

  - The level of community resources available.

    The need for accommodation (especially sheltered, eg staffed hostels, adult fostering) was often highlighted. It was sometimes necessary to keep people in hospital longer than necessary or to discharge them to unsuitable accommodation if an appropriate home could not be found for them. Discharging people to unsuitable accommodation could lead to relapse. Other resources frequently mentioned as lacking were day hospitals, day care centres and community staff (CPNs, social workers, occupational therapists)

  - Consideration of the full range of options

  - Time available in ward rounds for planning

  - The stage at which community staff were involved

  - Disagreements about who should provide care

- CPA was not commonly believed to affect discharge decisions, i.e to cause patients to remain in hospital because of a lack of community resources. Discharge decisions were often influenced by the demand for hospital beds; Where beds were in short supply patients may have to be discharged and, where they were not, patients could remain in hospital for longer.

- Responsibility for administration and communication lay mostly with ward staff and sometimes with medical staff. This placed extra demands on staff time and could take time away from patient care. Ward clerks were employed in one area to fulfil this role.

- The keyworker was appointed in the multi-disciplinary meeting. The selection of a keyworker was intended to be based on patient needs but this did not always happen. It could depend, for example, on which professions were present at the multi-disciplinary meeting.

- The keyworker was usually the person who would have the most contact with the patient once they were discharged. The role commonly fell to CPNs and social workers although CPNs reported that they were expected to take on the role more often than their social work colleagues. Consultants or other doctors could be the keyworker if they were seeing the patient regularly at out-patients. Day hospital staff, health visitors, care assistants and staff of residential homes were less often appointed keyworker. Voluntary agency workers, GPs and carers were not taking on this role.

CHAPTER 6 # Delivering the Care Plan in the Community

Once a patient had been discharged from hospital, the emphasis moved to the community side of the service. The logistics of delivering the planned care in the community had, on the whole, received less attention from those planning and operating CPA than the hospital based aspects.

This chapter looks at the role of the keyworker and the systems in place for reviewing care plans. Some of the factors affecting delivery of care plans are also discussed here. Finally, the impact of care planning on individual patients is considered.

6.1 The Keyworker's Role

The role of the keyworker had not been set out in detail in any of the CPA policy documents. Those planning for CPA had expected it to become defined as implementation proceeded and to be based on the needs of the patient. As keyworkers were appointed and more patients were discharged from hospital with a care plan, the keyworker's role had, out of necessity, evolved. With the lack of central guidance, each element of the community services had developed their own definition. This was often based on the service that they, as CPNs or social workers for example, had provided for people on their caseload prior to the implementation of CPA. It often did not differ markedly from previous practice. The definition was usually informal but sometimes recorded as part of the operational policy for a particular area of the service.

The main elements of a keyworker's role were identified as;

- Contributing to assessment and care planning while the patient is in hospital

- Keeping in contact with the patient once they are in the community

- Keeping in contact with other services involved

- Co-ordinating the planned services

- Working to prevent readmission

- Convening review meetings

Each of these elements is discussed in more detail below. In addition to these, keyworkers usually also provided a service specific to their own profession, for example, monitoring medication if a CPN.

Contributing to assessment and care planning prior to discharge

Keyworkers were appointed as part of the assessment procedure while the patient was still in hospital. Ideally they then attended one or more subsequent ward rounds or discharge planning meetings to contribute to planning. They might also visit the ward to get to know the patient and the other people involved in their care. It was reported, however, that this did not always happen and, in some cases, patients did not meet their keyworker until just before they left hospital, or even after leaving. It appeared that a lack of CPN and social work resources, coupled with historically weak links between the hospital and the community, contributed to this.

Keeping in contact and spending time with the patient

"He's (keyworker) available to talk to and pretty understanding and goes out of his way to try and help you if you are stuck with anything" (Carer)

Providing a point of contact with the mental health services, spending time with, and making active attempts to keep in touch with the patient and carer was an essential element of the keyworkers role. Regular visits had often been an established part of the keyworkers role as a community worker, for example a CPN or social worker. Thus being a "keyworker" did not require any alteration to this practice.

Users and carers placed great emphasis on keeping in contact when describing the keyworker's role. They spoke of the value of having a keyworker;

- To get in touch with at any time; a name and telephone number as a first point of contact.

- To provide a link with the mental health services once the patient has left hospital and thus counter feelings of isolation in the community.

- To talk to about any difficulties experienced, to let off steam, to help them think things through.

    "If you have got any personal or emotional problems it is good to be able to talk to them. Your head is so filled with all the problems and your illness that you can't see things clearly. They (keyworker) look at it from a different angle and can suggest the best way around it" (Ex-patient)

Users and carers reported widely differing degrees of input from their keyworkers. This ranged from the keyworker visiting once or twice a week, to visiting only when asked to do so or very infrequently. This was influenced by a number of factors;

- *The needs of the user and/or carer.*

Some found they required a very high level of input, especially when going through a difficult time. For others such constant contact was unnecessary;

    "I'm probably different from a lot of people... I don't need continuing support, most of the year I can manage perfectly well on my own, its only that (CPN) likes to monitor me if he knows that I'm going under any sort of

stress or anything. I can always ring and leave a message if he isn't there and he will come and see me. So we leave it like that most of the time" (Ex-patient, manic depression)

- *Keyworker caseload.*

In some parts of the service, rehabilitation units for example, the caseload was commonly relatively manageable, allowing the keyworker to give more input.

> *"If I am the keyworker for someone I give them more time. I spend time doing specific interventions with them but I might also provide support in quite a social way and they can contact me whenever they want. I'll give them my number so they can contact me when I'm available. That's not ideal because I am not here all the time. So it (keyworker role) is slightly more than doing interventions. Its really being there for them and giving them support and getting to know them as well"* (Occupational therapist, rehabilitation team).

Where caseloads were larger, however, there was not always time to spend in the above manner. Some users were aware that their keyworker was under pressure in this way. For example, one ex-patient felt that his keyworker had cancelled a number of appointments with him due to pressure of work. Another was reluctant to telephone the keyworker, knowing that many other people also had calls on their time.

- *Variations in approach to the keyworker role*

Sometimes the approach to the keyworker role varied between individuals. This could lead to a marked difference in the type and amount of input if the keyworker was replaced.

Where the keyworker role was taken by ward staff, day centre staff or consultants, keeping in contact was likely to be a less active process, relying on the patient to keep appointments at the hospital. If a patient did not attend, a further appointment would be given or arrangements made for community staff to visit.

- *Changes in keyworker role over time*

Some users and carers had found that their keyworker had initially been very enthusiastic and there had been frequent visits. As time had gone on, however, interest had appeared to wane and input dropped off; appointments were missed or not made. This unplanned withdrawal of service could leave the user or carer feeling let down.

Keeping in contact with the other services involved

It was recognised that effective care planning involved good communication between the various relevant parties.

"From my point of view it means that I have regular contact with the patient but it also means that I have to continuously feed back to everybody involved. And should a patient start breaking down it is on my shoulders and at the same time, I have to make sure that the others who are involved feed back to me and make it clear that I have got to be the person who is really on top of everything, because if the person starts to break down it is up to me to start arranging a domiciliary visit or whatever. Its using an awful lot of time writing an awful lot of letters and making a lot of phone calls just ensuring that the system with different professionals doesn't break down, let alone the patient. There are a lot of meetings to go to" (CPN)

Communication did not always happen smoothly, however. For example, the professionals involved in the plan sometimes did not keep the keyworker informed of developments. Problems in keeping in touch were exacerbated when those concerned were not based at the same location.

One carer had noticed that the social worker, occupational therapist and consultant did not keep in contact with each other in connection with her schizophrenic son, other than at case conferences. She commented that communication had been good initially but she now felt that the professionals were *"getting bored with it"*.

Co-ordinating the planned services

Co-ordination of other services in terms of making sure that the patient received all the elements of the care package was often mentioned as part of the keyworker's role. Sometimes, however, it appeared that the keyworkers themselves provided the majority of care in the community. In such cases co-ordination did not play much, if any, part..

It was important to strike a balance between providing care and the co-ordinating role. One health service manager felt that CPNs tended to take on more of a provision role as they were used to having to do everything themselves. They needed to learn to manage care programmes more generally.

In order to co-ordinate the services of other professionals it was necessary for the keyworker to have the authority to make sure that services were delivered. For example a CPN keyworker may not be able to make sure that a social worker or night sitter visits. All that they can do if input from these sources is not forthcoming is to refer to the management of the various services. In addition, some services could only be accessed through one "gate keeper", for example, it may be necessary for a social worker to arrange access to social services day, residential or respite care. Non-social services keyworkers would not be able to do this themselves. To date, it appeared that the issue of the level of authority implicit in the keyworker role had received little discussion.

In some cases it appeared that the keyworker was not expected to co-ordinate care as part of their role. For example, a day centre may appoint keyworkers for their clients who may also have a social worker and be attending out-patients. Here keyworking took place only in relation to the day centre services only and did not involve co-ordination with social work or medical staff. A lack of links between different community services was felt to contribute to this situation. Keyworking was sometimes seen as relating to just one aspect of the patient's care, for example, medication or housing.

Talking to users and carers showed that the keyworker also had a role in promoting awareness of community services and making suggestions where he or she felt that the client might take advantage of these. In this way users or carers had access to services that were not discussed prior to discharge. Sometimes the keyworker helped the user or carer to gain access to the services.

Preventing readmission

In some cases the keyworker role, along with the planned programme of care in the community, had been seen to be effective in preventing readmission to hospital.

> *"The care programme approach has enabled us to provide a system that, along with the stability of my staff and the view that we have of mental health, of preventing hospital admission and therefore I think we provide a better quality of service"* (Social services manager)

> *"It (following up people in the community as keyworker) saves me a lot of problems in the long run because, one, I get the patients earlier and resolve problems sooner and plus they are not back for relapse to give me hassle when they are on the ward. So it is to my advantage... Because we are so pressured to find beds for people I would rather find the problems earlier and be able to deal with them in the community, rather than have them as in-patients"* (Ward Manager, acute ward, acts as community keyworker to some patients)

> *"I know one lady who it has worked very well for - she has had 4 admissions in three years and she came out in February this year. On previous occasions she didn't have pre-discharge planning or follow-up. What had happened was that she was discharged and then a referral was sent through to the team which sometimes takes two weeks to get there, and by the time you have identified someone and actually got out there could be a months gap which, for this woman, was fatal. What she would do was that she would get better, she would go home. She would take her tablets for about two weeks and then say `Why am I taking tablets? I'm feeling great. I don't really need them so I'll stop taking them.' And within two weeks she was on a slope and even if you brought the tablets back you couldn't stop her. And she tried to do this the last time as well and the husband tried to feed her the tablets. So it was a matter of supporting the husband and educating the client; telling her why she was on tablets and why she had to take them. I supported her all through the time when she didn't want to take them any more and took her right through. She is doing remarkably well... she's firing*

on all cylinders. But if she stopped taking her tablets she would be back in hospital - there is no doubt" (CPN)

A number of professionals, however, pointed out that there were some cases for whom, due to the nature of their illness, relapse and readmission to hospital were almost inevitable, even given the best care planning. While CPA could not keep such cases out of hospital, it could affect their experience of hospitalisation in other ways. For example, closer monitoring in the community could mean that admission to hospital came about before a crisis rather than in response to one. In one area some such cases were admitted to the rehabilitation unit rather than the acute ward, thus avoiding one stage of the in-patient process.

> *"They are on somebody's caseload, they are falling down a bit, and instead of going straight onto an acute ward and then back to us they come straight to us... There was one who had had a domestic row with his family at home, needed somewhere to go so we took him in for respite. He was a client previously known to us and rather than go through the procedure of being admitted to the acute ward and picking up the habits and whatever there we took him into (rehabilitation unit) and he stayed a month. Now he is back out and the crisis is over. So by having the discharge and review meetings the community keyworker was able to say 'Hold on, I want him admitting'"* (Health service manager, rehabilitation)

Earlier intervention could also mean that the patient had to spend less time in hospital when they were readmitted.

> *"There is a lady I follow through... I co-ordinate her care and everything she wanted was available. But because of the nature of the illness she suffers she relapses and there is nothing whatsoever the services can do about that. And yet one of the consultants called the readmission a failure. I said `Why? She's not so bad this time and she'll require a far shorter period of hospitalisation this time because it has been picked up in its early stages.' It would have been a failure if she had just sat and festered"* (CPN)

Reviewing care

Keyworkers also had a responsibility in co-ordinating and providing input at review meetings (see Section 6.3)

A number of issues arose in relation to the keyworker role;

Changes in community staff roles since becoming keyworkers

Some CPNs, social workers, and other community staff commented that their roles had not changed since the keyworker system had been implemented. This was because they felt that they had been carrying out this role before or that it did not entail anything extra to their traditional roles. Others, however, believed that being a keyworker made one more responsible for the patient and for making sure that they had what was needed - it was not as easy to rely on other services as the keyworker had overall responsibility.

The role of the keyworker vs role of care manager

There was still some confusion as to whether care managers and keyworkers differed in their roles or not. Some professionals used the two terms interchangeably. In one particular area, however, there were both keyworkers and care managers. The differences between the two roles here were felt to be;

- *Client group*; Care managers had a lower caseload made up of people with more complex problems than that of a keyworker.

- *Type of intervention*; Keyworking involved shorter term intervention than care management and was often focused around specific tasks eg medication.

- *Distance from client*; Care managers would, in theory, be more distant from the client than a keyworker, taking a broker, rather than provider, role.

The situation was complicated, however, by the fact that one CPN or social worker could be a keyworker for some patients and a care manager for others. In addition care managers in this area were playing a major role in the delivery of care, while their role as brokers was not yet fully developed.

Continuity of care between the hospital and the community

Although the focus of CPA was initially on existing in-patients, some commented that its wider aim should be to provide continuity of service for clients moving between the hospital and the community.

> *"If we can change our focus so that, from the day you actually pick up a case, be it a GP referral that may need to go into in-patients, you're starting a CPA from there. In order to maintain this person's mental health state, the CPA collaboratively would indicate a period of admission, it is followed through by the same person so CPA is continual"* (Health service manager, acute services)

In practice, however, it was said that CPA plans did not always follow patients as they moved from acute to continuing care wards or acute wards to day hospital for example. Sometimes communication between hospital and community did not work smoothly so that, for instance, a CPN was not being given enough notice of discharge to be able to arrange services such as meals on wheels.

Resources required to carry out keyworker role

As well as needing extra time to provide a service to an increasing caseload, CPA also required keyworkers to spend more time in meetings, administration and communication.

CPA could increase the number of patients requiring community keyworkers and this put pressure on the workloads of CPNs and social workers in particular. Often these groups were already overstretched. Where this was the case the result could be that CPNs or social workers were:

- Unable or unwilling to take on the keyworker role.

    "There is that thought 'Oh, I don't want to be the keyworker because that is another person on my caseload and I am responsible'. There is that feeling that you are very responsible. You are a keyworker, you've got to take on all the co-ordination and the reviews as well. You have to plan the reviews and you have to get everyone together for the reviews which is quite a lot of work. Sometimes I think 'Do I want to be the keyworker here?'" (Occupational therapist, rehabilitation)

    "The capacity for social work on a provision basis under CPA is pretty remote" (Social services manager)

- Forced to limit the length of time for which they could fulfil the keyworker role for patients.

- Forced to discharge someone from their caseload before taking someone else on.

- Forced to limit the level of input they had with patients, for example only having time for the occasional visit.

6.2 Reviewing the Care Plan

The care programme approach requires regular reviews of the care plan while the client continues to live in the community. The three authorities in which CPA implementation had gone ahead were at differing stages in terms of whether reviews were taking place.

In one area reviews happened regularly in the rehabilitation and day centre services. These parts of the service had always had a review process but this was now formalised using the CPA paperwork. In the acute service reviews were also reported to be taking place, although perhaps not as frequently as expected. In the EMI wards a review procedure was to be implemented in the near future. In this area reviews were felt to be important because:

- They were useful in monitoring the patient's progress.

- They allowed professionals to check that patients were receiving the services planned and using them appropriately.

- People may agree to a plan of aftercare when they are in hospital in order to be allowed to leave and then want it changed once they are in the community.

- While the person is an in-patient it may be difficult to identify what their needs might be in the community. The pre-discharge care plan can then be seen as a starting point and modified during the review procedure.

The remaining two areas still had work to do in establishing their review procedure. Reviews were not taking place here except for those patients who had a care manager, were subject to Section 117 of the Mental Health Act 1983, or had been discharged from a specialist rehabilitation unit. Implementation was said to be held back by both the lack of a computerised system to cope with prompting review and a need to overcome difficulties in getting people together for a review.

Convening reviews

It was intended that the initial review date be set prior to discharge in the multi-disciplinary meeting. This was sometimes not possible, for example where a keyworker had not been appointed by this time. It was generally the responsibility of the keyworker or care manager to call subsequent reviews. In some cases, however, the consultant or ward manager had taken on this role. One consultant set aside a particular time to review patients and the other parties had to fit in with this.

Timeframe

In the area where reviews were taking place, the time frame specified by the CPA policy was around three months initially and thereafter as often as required. It appeared that staff were aware of this timetable and that reviews were taking place accordingly. The keyworker could call an earlier review if there was a crisis or, alternatively, decide not to call a review if there seemed to be no need. The rehabilitation unit here had traditionally held reviews every six weeks and continued to do so.

Communication

Communication was of vital importance to the review procedure. Ideally all parties needed to be informed of the date and time of the review and reminded to attend. This did not always happen in practice, however. One of the reasons for this was that the responsibility for such communication usually lay with the keyworker who may not have sufficient time or administrative support to consistently fulfil this role. In each area the need for a system, preferably computerised, designed to "flag up" reviews was acknowledged and there were plans to move in this direction. At present it was up to the keyworker to remember to organise the review. This could be difficult when the keyworker was not sent a copy of the care plan, which was sometimes the case.

> *"There are operational issues that we didn't address when we were planning... it's lost to posterity (care plan is put on file) until the next time in hospital... one hopes that the keyworker knows and remembers that it was agreed that the next case conference would be on the next date or in three months time and it was their responsibility to try and co-ordinate consultants and all the other people having to come to case conferences - it's quite difficult for some of them"* (Social services manager)

Multi-disciplinary working in reviews

Although it was generally acknowledged that reviews should involve all of the professions that were relevant, the extent to which this happened in practice varied.

When someone was discharged from a rehabilitation unit or to care management a wider range of professionals was likely to attend the review. This appeared to be due to the strength of existing team working or review procedures and the efforts made to involve a large number of people. It was possible that patients in such units by definition required a greater range of involvement. Reviews here could involve community staff (CPNs, social workers etc), the consultant, the patient and relatives. Hospital staff were not commonly involved.

At the other extreme were reviews taking place at out-patients, in which just the doctor, not necessarily a consultant, and the patient were present. Sometimes input from CPNs, social workers or other community staff was sought.

> *"What happens is that, when I see them in out-patients I would then be asking the community nurse to join me. That is virtually what a review meeting is"* (Consultant, acute)

This consultant pointed out, however, that in his experience the keyworker rarely attended the review unless there was a problem to be sorted out.

Where patients came into CPA straight from the community, reviews would be held with the appropriate parties, for example the GP, the patient and the social worker/CPN.

If the review had been called in response to a crisis situation there were likely to be fewer people involved.

The need for separate meetings

There was some confusion as to whether a full multi-disciplinary meeting was necessary to review the aftercare plan. Some felt that this was too much of an undertaking.

> *"If you are going to call a meeting every six months as you are supposed to then that involves a lot of people getting together to discuss things - a lot of arrangements. So there is a lot of administration time needed to call an additional meeting like that. And there are a lot of folks sitting around*

spending a lot of time discussing one individual whereas most of us feel that, since there is so much demand on our time, it is better to get on with the job and spend 10 minutes on half a dozen people... then in that way we at least have an input on a wider range... That is why I am trying to get an atmosphere of continual monitoring, supervision, multi-disciplinary discussion of patients who are involved with the services - so a regular discussion of everyone involved with a keyworker... and doing it relatively informally rather than having a special meeting that you call together and sit everyone down... If you have called everyone together things tend to go on a bit, everyone wants their say and the meetings that we have had have gone on for an hour and a half or two hours for an individual client - that is a bit excessive when you have got lots of other people" (Consultant, acute)

In one area, the mental health manager did not see a full case conference as necessary but believed that some of his staff did and were daunted by this.

Reviews at out-patients could be rushed due to a busy timetable. There was a case for holding separate meetings, although these could be difficult to convene.

"It does feel better if you are going along specifically for a community discharge and aftercare review and not rushing through a clinic as well. Because (in a separate meeting) the focus is more on the patient and their functioning; how is the whole thing working?, what is needed?, what is working?, what isn't working?, and the CPN and the social worker will be there" (CPN, acute)

Recording

In all areas there were forms on which to record the date & outcome of a review. In the area where reviews were happening it was said that these forms were not always filled in, as the appropriate documents were not always available.

Discharge from CPA

There was some debate and confusion as to whether CPA was an ongoing process, or whether patients could be discharged from it. Primarily this revolved around whether the patient might be discharged from the keyworker's caseload. Acute patients were generally believed to need follow-up for a shorter time than people with longer term illnesses who may need it indefinitely. There was a danger, however, in discharging patients who appeared to be doing well in the community but who may then have a crisis and have no keyworker keeping in contact regularly. On the other hand, a heavy workload for community staff could necessitate discharge from caseloads. For one community mental health team CPA had meant following up more people for a shorter time.

"What we have guaranteed is that everyone who is allocated a keyworker must have a review within three months and that review will then have to

establish whether we need to do further work or not. So, for example, a carer who has had someone diagnosed with dementia 18 months ago; he had linked into support groups and has got services going in and really the role was really just a link between that person and the team and going out to check that they are fine. Or perhaps the carer, every two months, needed to offload. I'm saying, `Sorry, but if I'm having to prioritise that is the sort of thing that is going to have to go at the moment'" (Health service manager)

Users' and carers' experiences of reviews

Very few of the users or carers interviewed had been involved in a review meeting since the time of discharge from hospital, or knew of any plans to hold one. Where reviews had taken place, all the relevant professionals had not necessarily been present. In one case there had been a review meeting 6 weeks after the patient had left hospital. The social worker and consultant had been unable to attend. The CPN and patient did attend and arranged to meet again at a later date and the social worker sent a letter to the meeting saying that social work input would no longer be provided. In another case it was left to the carer to ask for meetings with the occupational therapist, consultant and relatives of the patient when she felt it necessary. A case conference, organised by social services, did, however, take place every six months as there was a child involved.

6.3 Implications of Care Plans for Users and Carers

The focus of this research was on the process of care planning rather than the content and delivery of the care plans themselves. The study did not set out to evaluate the impact of CPA on the community care of people with mental illness. However, during the course of the study some information was gathered, from ex-patients and carers and professionals, about the nature and effect of care plans. This is briefly described here. More thorough investigation and a differently designed study would be needed to assess fully the impact of the CPA initiative on the quality of care in the community.

Nature of care plans

The care plans developed varied widely in complexity from one or two out-patients appointments to a complex plan with a range of input from a number of sources. Three examples are given below illustrating first simple, and then more complex, care plans. These are care plans as described by patients and carers interviewed;

> Mr G is 49 and, for many years, has had periods when he is very anxious and worried. He has been admitted to hospital on several occasions. He lives with his wife in their own home. They have a CPN who visits around once a month. He talks to them both,

explains about the drugs that Mr G needs to take and persuades him to keep taking them (he has stopped in the past and had to be readmitted to hospital). The CPN also provides a point of contact with the hospital services and Mrs G finds this particularly helpful. Apart from an out-patients appointment every three months to review Mr G's medication they feel that they need no further help.

Mrs C is 80 and suffers from dementia. She is cared for at home by her husband. A member of the community mental health team acts as their keyworker and a worker from the local community centre has also been very helpful and is a point of contact. The keyworker has helped them with a number of activities including applying for benefits, visiting a residential home with a view to providing respite and perhaps full time care in the longer term, and helping them with their banking arrangements. Mr C prefers to care for Mrs C at home while this is possible and finds the help of the keyworker and community centre worker very useful. He counts them as friends and can telephone them whenever he needs to. Often, however, they telephone her first.

"I've promised them that I wouldn't go through any stress or worry, they're there when I need them... I can honestly say that the care Mrs G has had in the hospital and since she has been home is first class, they are not leaving a stone unturned"

Mrs D is a carer for her 25 year old daughter (K) who has schizophrenia. K lives nearby with her young son and relies on her parents very much. They often look after their grandson, sometimes for days at a time. K sees her consultant every three weeks and a CPN comes once a fortnight to give injections. They would like further support from the CPN but their doctor has told them that this is not available. A social worker has been involved for a number of years and will visit if asked. Mrs D feels that the social worker is supposed to be the keyworker but she does not have any input unless in an emergency. K also has an occupational therapist who visits for a couple of weeks if called in. Mrs D would like to see counselling offered to her son-in-law and more practical input from the social worker and occupational therapist.

Changes in discharge planning and aftercare

Users and carers with a history of hospital admissions were asked whether they had observed any changes in discharge planning or aftercare received since the implementation of CPA. Responses ranged from those who had noticed no difference at all to some who felt that their aftercare had improved.

One patient who suffered from depression, for example, commented that when he was first ill (prior to CPA implementation) he had had no follow-up on discharge from hospital, although he could not cope with his finances. More recently (after CPA implementation) he has had back-up care; someone to talk to and to fall back on in times of stress. He felt that talking with this person, his care manager, would help him to avoid being admitted to hospital when he became depressed.

Another patient, who suffered from paranoid psychosis, had found that he now had a far more comprehensive care plan than previously;

> *"Before when I used to leave hospital they used to just send me to the doctor to make sure that I got my medication and that was mainly it"*

This person now had a keyworker (social worker) who was helping him with a consumer rights issue, out-patients appointments, a CPN (arranging for him to get help with cooking), someone to help him buy new furniture when he moved into a flat. In addition some social contact was being arranged through the MIND befriending service.

It is interesting to note, however, that people who had experienced an improvement in aftercare had either been discharged from a rehabilitation ward or to care management. Patients discharged from acute wards with a keyworker had not observed any such differences. One ex-patient, who suffered from manic depression and had recently been in an acute ward, had noted that there was now a definite procedure in discharge planning meetings and paperwork to accompany it. This, however, had not had an impact on the actual aftercare received.

> *"If I hadn't known what was going on I would have been quite baffled... It was explained to me, the CPN said there were new procedures. It all sounded like lip service, like `This is something we have to do'... They all had these sheets of things to go through... It didn't seem any different to me than the last time. I had just as good care last time as I have this time... They were all signing things and agreeing to do things... having it all down in writing, but that's what happened anyway last time"* (Ex-patient)

6.4 Summary

Keyworker role

- The role of the keyworker had not been formally set out in detail, but had evolved based on existing community staff roles.

- The main elements of the keyworker's role were felt to be:

  - Contributing to assessment and care planning prior to discharge

  - Keeping in contact/spending time with the user or carer

  - Keeping in contact with other services

  - Co-ordinating planned services

  - Preventing readmission

  - Reviewing care

- There was some confusion as to how the roles of keyworker and care manager differed.

- One of the aims of care planning was to provide continuity of care between the hospital and community. This did not, however, always happen in practice.

- Extra staff resources were required to carry out the keyworker role. More patients were being referred to keyworkers, there were more meetings to attend and more administration and communication was required. Community staff were usually already overstretched and resource limitations could mean that they were unable or unwilling to take on the keyworker role, forced to limit the amount of time or input they could devote to the role or forced to discharge some patients from their caseload in order to take others on.

Review

- Authorities were at differing stages with their implementation of review procedures. In one area, reviews were happening in most services, although not comprehensively. In the other two authorities where CPA had been implemented there was still work to be done on establishing the review procedure. This had been held back by the absence of a computerised system for prompting reviews and a need to overcome difficulties in getting those involved together.

- It was intended that the review date be set at the multi-disciplinary meeting but this did not always happen. It was generally the responsibility of the keyworker to call subsequent reviews, either at set intervals or as needed.

- Communication was very important in terms of informing relevant people of the date and time of the review. Often this was the keyworker's responsibility and they may have little time for administration. It was hoped that a computerised system for flagging up reviews would facilitate better communication.

- Reviews were likely to involve more professionals in rehabilitation services. Here they commonly involved community staff, the user, relatives, consultant and other relevant parties. At the other extreme, some reviews were held with just the consultant and the patient present. There was some confusion as to whether a separate meeting was required or whether reviews could take place at an out-patients appointment.

- Forms had been designed to record reviews taking place and their outcomes.

- There was some debate as to whether CPA was designed to be ongoing or whether people could be discharged from it. Keyworker workload could play a role here; if resources were stretched keyworkers may have to work with more people but for a shorter time.

Implications of Care Plans for Users and Carers

- This study has not addressed the effect of CPA on the care plans devised or the outcome for users and carers. However some information of this nature was gathered. Some users with a history of hospital admissions had found that their aftercare had improved since the implementation of CPA. Others had not observed any change.

CHAPTER 7   Working Together

It was acknowledged that collaboration was necessary at a number of levels for the care programme approach to work effectively on a day to day basis;

- Ground level staff from health and social services need to discuss assessment and care planning and to keep in touch with each other to monitor patients' care in the community.

- Users and carers need to be aware of and in agreement with the plans made, so consultation with them is important.

- Voluntary agencies should be involved in care planning and in the delivery of care where appropriate.

Assessment and discharge planning meetings were commonly attended by the patient, the consultant and/or other doctors, and ward staff. In many cases CPNs, social workers and relatives of the patient would also attend. Occupational therapists, psychologists and day hospital staff were less likely to be there unless they were a member of an existing team. Equally, staff from voluntary agencies, housing departments, etc, were not consistently involved, and this was a source of some concern. General practitioners were not often involved, although in one acute unit GPs did sometimes attend discharge planning meetings. In rehabilitation and long stay units meetings were likely to involve more professionals as a wider range of staff usually took part in team working.

This chapter looks at the extent to which health professionals, social workers, users and carers, and voluntary agencies are involved in CPA. The factors which may make involvement difficult are identified and any plans for overcoming these highlighted.

7.1 Collaboration between Statutory Agency Staff

The care programme approach often necessitated the input of more than one profession, both in assessment and care planning and in the delivery of care in the community. This was not usually an entirely new way of working; in some cases teams comprising a relatively large number of disciplines were already in existence, while in others working practices had changed so that a wider range of people was now involved.

Working in this way raised a number of issues surrounding the logistics of convening and attending multi-disciplinary meetings, links between hospital and community and between health and social services.

Multi-disciplinary meetings usually took place as part of an established ward round, although more disciplines may now be involved. For example, where a profession had previously received a referral, they may now be invited to attend a meeting. On the whole, attendance at these meetings was felt to be useful, with more emphasis now being placed on discharge planning.

> *"It has made other people in the team recognise planning a bit more. A lot of planning went on by certain people in the team but there was a need to look a bit wider at all the issues. You would have a medical person having someone into hospital and saying, `OK, this person is depressed, hallucinating, deluded... We are going to take them into hospital and assess the situation, we are going to give them this medication and OK all the symptoms are gone now.' And once they (consultant) have finished they look at you and say, 'By the way, how about the home situation?' - that could have happened in the past but it's making everybody more aware that we need to start from the beginning"* (Ward manager)

A number of factors influenced the effectiveness of multi-disciplinary working;

Time needed to attend meetings

> *"The will is there but they (CPN service and social workers) just don't have the people"* (Consultant, acute)

Attending hospital based ward rounds was time consuming and competing demands on professionals' time often made it difficult for them to attend. The problem was compounded for staff based at other sites who needed to travel to meetings. In addition, some community staff, for example district based social workers, did not deal exclusively with mental illness. Their time could be prioritised towards other areas, such as child protection, thus making it even more difficult to find time to attend aftercare meetings. Hospital based staff such as psychologists and occupational therapists, who only had time to see a limited number of clients, also found it difficult to allocate time to attend meetings.

Further difficulties arose when community staff were allocated to clients within specified geographical sectors, while wards and consultants within the hospital were not organised in this way. This meant that a CPN or social worker may have patients in a number of wards, and under the care of a number of consultants. Thus they may need to attend several ward rounds each week in order to discuss all of their patients. CPNs in one such area had initially been invited to all CPA meetings. Because of time constraints they had been unable to attend and it had been necessary for ward staff to carry out some screening so that CPNs were not invited in every case.

Attending ward rounds was made easier where there was a set timetable determining when each patient was discussed. It was then possible to attend the meeting for that period of time only, rather than sitting through discussions relating to a number of patients. In some wards, this type of system was in operation but its success depended on consultants adhering to the timetable set. There had been occasions when people had turned up for a meeting at the appointed time to find that the case had already been discussed or that they had to wait.

Social workers had been able to be involved in discussing care plans in one area as they had a regular short meeting with the consultant especially for this purpose. This was a compromise arrived at because the social workers did not have the time to attend the longer ward rounds.

Logistics of convening meetings.

The number of people who might be involved in a case could make it difficult to convene a meeting.

> "If you get both a CPN and a social worker to attend you are very fortunate because there is usually one of them who will ring and say `I'm afraid I can't make it at that time, can you arrange it for a different time?' And you can't because the consultant has only got that particular morning to do it in so it makes life very hard sometimes" (Ward staff, acute ward)

> "This is a case we discharged about three months ago. We had a lady come to us with a chronic depressive illness....she was a diabetic on insulin twice a day, she was also a stroke person and had a fractured femur.....she had a district nurse going in for the insulin, she had to have a CPN to manage the psychiatric monitoring, she had a person to go and manage her home, there was physiotherapy involved, district dietician. Now if you are discharging that person you fill in a piece of paper. Sometimes all these people haven't got the luxury of time to synchronise mutually and all sit there and fill in their bits" (Ward manager,)

There could be reluctance on the part of some professions to become involved despite repeated requests from the convener. This was a criticism often made of social workers by other professionals. Where there were both hospital and community based social workers this problem was sometimes reported to stem from conflict as to which type of social worker would become involved.

Communication

Communication was of key importance in multi-disciplinary working, particularly in terms of making sure that the relevant people were aware of the time and place of meetings. Sometimes community staff were not even made aware that their client had been admitted to hospital. A number of factors influenced how effectively such communication took place;

- Awareness by consultant or ward staff of professions already involved with the patient. Sometimes a degree of detective work was required to establish who the relevant people in the community were.

> "For instance today I have tried to arrange an aftercare meeting for one patient. I rang the social work district office for the area that she lives in only to be told `Oh well, that lady has her own social worker because she

actually lives in a community home' so you say `Thank you very much'. Then you ring the community home and they say `Oh yes, she's out at the moment but I'll get her to call you back.' Then it was `She might not be able to attend but we can send somebody else.' So you still don't know who is actually coming to that meeting and that's only for one patient. Then you ring the CPN and they say `We don't actually think we can input anything but if you do really need us to come we'll send someone.' Now that, in my book, is not really a satisfactory attitude to aftercare' (Ward staff, acute)

- Efficiency in inviting people to meetings, for example by sending letters. This can depend on the level of clerical resources available or the time available to non-clerical staff to carry out clerical work. A number of staff commented that they had not been invited to meetings where they felt they should have been.

- Giving sufficient notice of the meeting for people to attend.

  "Its run in such a hotch potch way that it is decided just one or two days before and we have done our diaries four weeks ahead" (Member of CMHT)

- Mechanisms for informing those involved when meetings have been cancelled or are not running to schedule; Administration systems did not always take such situations into account.

Deciding who is to be involved in the multi-disciplinary process

It was generally the responsibility of the consultant and/or ward staff to decide who should be invited to CPA meetings. For example, it could be decided that the input of a certain profession was not necessary or that certain staff are too busy to be involved. The attitudes of individual consultants towards joint working could affect the extent to which other professions were involved; some consultants liked to work in teams, whereas others preferred to work more on their own. At the latter extreme, it was reported that a consultant and ward nurse completed the CPA paperwork themselves after deciding that no-one else was needed.

Sometimes a degree of selectivity on the part of ward staff and consultants was useful to professionals, enabling them to better organise their time. However, some felt that they would rather do their own assessment to determine which patients they should be involved with. A psychologist, for example, felt that he could quickly determine which patients needed his input by going onto the wards. Instead, it was up to the consultants to refer cases to him.

In one area it was reported that some professions were attending CPA meetings because they believed that this was required of them, rather than because they were going to be involved with a patient. There was concern that this was wasting time.

Provisions where there is non-attendance of key professionals

Some provisions were made to cope with situations when people necessary to the care plan had not been present at the multi-disciplinary meeting. These included;

- Sending a copy of the plans made through the post.

- Postponing the meeting if it was vital to have the keyworker present or otherwise conveying the outcome to them

- Making a provisional care plan in the hope that the necessary staff would agree to it.

In some cases, however, it was reported that no consultation took place. For example, in one area there was a column on the CPA forms to record that, if someone could not attend, they had been consulted. This was not always completed.

Links between hospital and community

Multi-disciplinary working was easier when there were good links and channels for communication between hospital and community staff. In some cases these links were reported to be less than ideal, with community staff not having a strong presence on the wards. As one ward manager explained:

> "In X health authority the community team is alienated from the ward area altogether. I think its the way they practice in the service. All the patients they see have been in hospital, it would be easier for them if they came to see us and said `how is so and so?'. And we could give them feedback on how they are when they are ill and they could tell us how they are when they are well".

In another area, differing practices between consultants affected links between hospital and community services. One consultant had regular meetings with the community staff to discuss patients; another (in the same unit) had a much less formal system relying on the consultant or ward staff to choose which community staff were involved in discharge planning. Community staff felt that the latter scenario made care planning more 'hit and miss' and preferred a more structured approach.

It was important for effective care planning that barriers between hospital and community be broken down. Statutory requirements such as Section 117 (Mental Health Act 1983) aftercare were said to be contributing to this. To some extent CPA had helped to introduce more effective communication. For example, CPNs in one area were now more aware of other services involved. Before CPA was implemented they may not have known, for example, that a client of theirs was attending day hospital.

Links between community staff

The strength of collaboration, at ground level, between various professionals working in the community could also affect multi-disciplinary working. Communication was easier when multi-disciplinary and inter-agency teams were established in the community and based in one geographical location. Sometimes, however, the various community based professionals worked in relative isolation from each other. For example, a patient may have both a CPN and a social worker involved, with neither knowing what input the other is providing. This could lead to a duplication of care and render the co-ordination element of the keyworker role very difficult. In effect, the service users could find themselves with a number of keyworkers, none of whom were actually co-ordinating the care given.

Strategies for good multi-disciplinary working

Multi-disciplinary working in the community was felt to take place more smoothly under the following conditions;

-   Where all professionals are working together or regularly meeting together in one place, for example a community mental health team or multi-disciplinary ward round, so that interactive discussion can take place.

-   Where no one member of the team dominates.

-   Where the team is self contained with a defined client group and aims.

In one area the elderly services had implemented a "link worker" system to establish better communication between the hospital and community. Here one member of the community mental health team attended all ward rounds on a rotation basis and reported back to the team. This system had been instigated as keyworkers were not initially being appointed and invited to ward rounds. As the system became established, however, the link worker was able to ensure that a community keyworker was nominated and keyworkers were then able to attend ward rounds. Thus the link worker system was now, to some extent, becoming redundant, with both link and key workers attending ward rounds.

> "One person would come back to the team and would be able to say `Mrs So and So?, yes, I was there Tuesday. This is the reason why she is going to need a key worker. There is all this stuff involved that is going on that needs unscrambling and services going in'. So it means instead of a team just sitting with a... (CPA form) and saying 'Who is this woman?'.....they did actually know everybody....I think what has happened is that the guidelines about how someone actually gets a keyworker have actually started to work because link workers went to the ward rounds and started educating ward staff and vice versa and it has brought them closer together. So now the communication goes on naturally day by day without needing this enforced presence at a ward round to sort it out so often. By the time people get to the

ward round, the ward has already rung the team, the team have allocated a keyworker, the keyworker has been in touch and the link worker is sitting here saying, 'Well actually, I've got nothing to do anymore.'" (Manager, CMHT, EMI)

7.2 *Involvement of Users and Carers*

One of the key principles of CPA is the involvement of users and carers in the aftercare planning process. In three of the authorities the policy documents emphasised that this was expected;

> *"The patient, and carer, where appropriate, will be involved and fully informed regarding the patient's treatment and individual care plan... Interventions will be planned with the patient and carer, wherever possible, to ensure their understanding and involvement"*

> *"It is very important that patients and carers are involved in the discharge planning as far as possible. Every effort should be made to seek their wishes and agree and explain what plans have been made"*

> *"Assessment: A multi-disciplinary process to identify an individual's health and social care needs. Should closely involve patient, carer and indicate their views"*

> (Extracts from policy documents)

In all areas where CPA had been implemented there was widespread agreement with the principle of involving users and carers. This was felt to be "common sense" and necessary to ensure commitment to the care plan.

> *"We would like to fit it (care plan) to the client much more in order for the client to have some control over it and in order that it will work for them and they will have some commitment to it"* (Social worker)

A number of professionals pointed out that users and carers had traditionally been included in planning their aftercare, at least to the extent of seeking their agreement with plans made.

> *"I would hope that I had always involved carers as much as possible before this anyway. I have always made it a policy that carers are not just accepted, they are encouraged to attend the ward round and to discuss things there and if they are not going to do that then they are collared when they visit and if they don't turn up then we go out and make contact with them. So I think we are already doing what was intended. And if somebody needs to go home you can't sort of chuck people out and carers find their relatives are on the doorstep without them knowing about it - they have to be informed. They have to know what is going on and if they object to it then their voices are heard"* (Consultant, acute)

> *"There isn't any formal 'we have got to discuss this with the patient, tick a box and say that the patient agrees with this'. That might sound as if the patient is ignored in all that but whenever we are discussing and arranging*

things then the patient has to be involved in the discussions since they have got to take the tablets, they have got to attend, they have got to go home on weekend leave or what have you. For the most part it is a question of joint agreement; 'We think you ought to be taking these tablets, what do you feel about them?'. And if they refuse that is certainly taken into account. If you are planning on say a weekend leave for a patient - you think they are ready to go but not quite ready for discharge then you have to take their level of confidence into account - if they feel that they can't manage it then they aren't going to manage it" (Consultant, acute)

Instances were reported, however, both by users and carers and professionals, where patients were not present at discharge planning meetings or ward rounds.

Potential for users/carers to be involved in CPA

There were a number of levels at which users and carers could play a part in the CPA procedure. These ranged from passive acceptance of information to taking an active role in formulating the care plan;

- *Information* - Informing users and carers of rights to aftercare, of CPA policy and of plans made (in either verbal or written form).

- *Consent* - Obtaining users' and/or carers' agreement to having an aftercare programme, the programme planned, the involvement of relatives or carers and the information kept about them. Gaining carers' consent to their involvement in the care plan and carers' consent on behalf of the patient if illness makes it difficult for the patient to participate.

- *Consultation* - Providing opportunities for dialogue to find out patients' and carers' wishes in relation to care following discharge, and eliciting their reactions to care plans suggested.

Around half of the users and carers interviewed felt that they had been able to express their views in some form. These tended to have been patients in rehabilitation or EMI wards or discharged under a care management system. Some had been asked what they felt their needs were and how they would like them met. Others had been presented with a care plan and their agreement sought. Many were unaware that a formal "plan" of care had been formulated.

Forum for involvement

The forum for the above involvement was commonly a ward round or perhaps a separate discharge planning meeting. The majority of the users and carers interviewed reported attending multi-disciplinary meetings or ward rounds to discuss their aftercare. Review meetings were less commonly held.

A number of factors were said to influence whether or not users and carers attended such meetings;

- The nature of the mental illness could cause patients to forget to or be unwilling to attend. In contrast, ex-patients who were coping well in the community may not feel that they need to attend review meetings.

- Sometimes patients and carers were not invited to meetings. This could be due to patients being too ill to attend, a lack of communication, the attitudes of staff to involving patients and carers, or because the patient did not wish the carer or relative to be present.

- Sometimes the patient or carer did not wish to attend. For example, one carer did not want her schizophrenic son to be taken away from her but hospital staff had suggested in the past that he leave home. For this reason, she avoided meeting with the consultant. In other cases relatives and carers did not attend because they were not interested.

Expressing an opinion

Users and carers were most involved in CPA when they were encouraged to give their views on what services were needed and to take an active part in the formulation of the care plan. Such consultation, however, did not take place consistently. Although both the circular and the policy documents in two of the areas envisaged that it would happen, there were a number of factors which appeared to prevent it.

There were issues on which patients, carers and professionals did not always agree. For example;

- *Discharge decisions*

  The decision concerning whether and when to discharge the patient lay ultimately with the consultant. Although patients' and carers' views could be taken into account here, more often they were not. In many cases patients and carers were happy to leave this decision with the consultants, - feeling that they had the appropriate expertise. Sometimes, however, patients and carers felt that the period of hospitalisation should be extended or that the patient should be discharged earlier.

- *Details of the aftercare plan*

  "We had a patient who we wanted to discharge to a hostel and the patient agreed, but the relatives would not have it, so eventually we had to change the plan and allow the patient to go home which we thought was not very good for them. We had to give in... we thought to keep the good will and the support, because they were very supportive to the patient when he was at home and still it was not right because they were giving in to everything he was asking and we thought that a period in a hostel would be more appropriate for him to learn a bit more about living skills" (Ward manager, acute)

Sometimes this disagreement was voiced, but in other cases patients and carers were reluctant to put forward their point of view. There were a number of reasons for this;

- The threatening nature of ward rounds as a forum for consultation.

- Reluctance to "rock the boat" in case the discharge decision was affected.

- The influence of the mental illness/patient status itself.

The ward round as a forum for consultation

Although discharge and aftercare planning commonly took place in ward rounds, many professionals and users and carers felt that this was not the most appropriate setting. There were many reasons for this (see Chapter 5), one of which concerned their suitability as a forum in which patients could make a valid contribution.

The presence of a number of professionals could make expressing an opinion a daunting prospect for patients and carers;

> *"Ostensibly the opportunity is there because they are an equal part of the group - In practice, I think because it is a multi-disciplinary group, they feel overpowered and not able to contribute. Often people with mental illness have very low self esteem... and they are frightened of opening their mouth because it might sound stupid and there are all these "professionals" around them, discussing what should happen to them and sometimes it can be quite off-putting to break into that and say 'Well, look here, I'm not sure about that"* (Voluntary agency)

The formality of the ward round situation could make patients feel that they should play a particular role.

> *"I tried to play the part, be confident like them, confident and serious. Obviously I wasn't confident"* (Ex-patient)

Sometimes patients were not informed in advance about the nature of the meeting.

> *"When I was going there I didn't expect to be in a big room, it was a huge room with a lot of space in the middle and all these people round. And I went in and (thought) ... 'Is this what all the shrinks are doing? their tea break?'... I didn't know what it was... They said 'Dr A wants to see you', I was told by one nurse. He led me in through some kind of secret door... behind there was a little room... I thought I was not seeing a lot of people, I was amazed"* (Ex-patient, acute ward).

Finding out about the aftercare plans for the first time at the pre-discharge meeting could present an added pressure;

> *"What seems to be the problem on the wards is that the client does not get to see the form until the meeting and there seems to be no discussion between the keyworker and the client. I went to one (meeting) three weeks ago with a very vulnerable client and the ward staff had said to him; 'You have to agree to your discharge plan' and he felt that he was being frogmarched into this meeting to agree to do certain things. And the meeting went into a terrible state because he was so angry and we couldn't*

get him calmed down. It should have just been a discussion about what everyone was doing, but he felt that he was going to be made to do things he didn't want to" (CPN)

A number of alternative strategies for eliciting the views of patients and carers were suggested or already in place;

- *Reducing the number of people present at the meeting*

  One hospital unit asked patients how many people they would like present at the meeting. The aftercare plan would then be discussed between those professionals and the patient. Afterwards, if there was any disagreement with the proposed plan, the full group of professionals would again discuss the situation.

  One ex-patient described how he went to a meeting with around 10 people whom he didn't know. He was asked a lot of questions and just answered "yes" or "no". He felt that a meeting with the consultant and the keyworker would have been sufficient. This would have allowed for more discussion between himself and the professionals so that they had more information from which to formulate a care plan.

- *Keyworker meeting one to one with patient*

  It was suggested, in one area, that the keyworker meet with the patient on a one to one basis to discuss the care plans, and then feed back the patient's view at the ward round.

  In another area, an occupational therapist described how she made sure that, if she was the keyworker, she went over the decisions made in the multi-disciplinary meeting with the patient afterwards to make sure that they understood and agreed.

  > *"(I say to the patients) `In the meeting, you were there, we decided that I was to be your keyworker, is that OK?' (they usually say in the meeting that it is OK). And then I say, 'This is what we are going to concentrate on because this has been identified, do you agree that they are the main problem areas that we need to work on?'. And then I say 'If you need me I'm here. You can ring me whenever you feel you need to. If there is something that you are not sure about who you are going to see or what you are going to do ring me or come and see me'"* (Occupational therapist, rehabilitation)

- *Voluntary agencies as advocates*

  Some voluntary agencies suggested that they may be able to play a role as advocates in the ward round situation, either attending instead of the patient or carer and presenting their views, or accompanying the patient or carer to provide support.

  > *"If someone (from voluntary agency) went to that meeting armed with what the carers think needs to happen for their (patient) rather than for the professionals to sit down and say 'This, this and this, lets tell them', that would be an improvement. And in fact, I don't know what the size of the*

problem is, but ....(voluntary agency) for instance would be willing to act as advocates in those kind of circumstances" (Voluntary agency)

Voluntary agency workers with knowledge of the hospital systems, mental health issues and community care could act on behalf of the patient and carer in an assertive and informed manner. However, one carer had found that the health authority was reluctant to have a voluntary agency involved. The resource implications for such organisations would also need to be considered.

Reluctance to "rock the boat"

The priority for many patients was being allowed to leave hospital, a decision in the hands of those at the multi-disciplinary meeting. They were therefore anxious not to do anything which may lead to the hospital stay being lengthened. Some believed that expressing an opinion in the meeting could have this effect.

> *"There is perhaps a desire not to rock the boat in case the discharge doesn't go ahead - you have got to agree to these things because this is the only way they are going to be allowed out"* (Voluntary agency)

> *"I was called, they (professionals) were already sitting there. It seems that they were seeing other people as well. I was called in, in a big room, and they were all sitting in armchairs. My psychiatrist talked to me and he asked me how I was and everything, and things like that. You see, I was very fragile because I didn't want to go to hospital again (ie stay in hospital). So I had to be very quiet, to tell them that I was very calm ... and not pressure them to discharge me. Because if you pressure them ... they object to it (ie to being discharged)... I was just very calm and everything they said; I agreed. Because if you say 'Oh, I want to go home, definite', that's it, full stop, they'll never let you go home because they always say the opposite of what you want"* (Ex-patient)

> *"When your position is so shakey and you are either out or in, it is like a prison. You don't want to be there, you can't be demanding and asking, because you just want to.. (go home).. You're like a mouse"* (Ex-patient)

Influence of the nature of mental illness/patient status on ability to participate in consultation

Often the mental illness itself led to apathy and low self-esteem, which made it difficult for patients to express their opinions.

> *"There tends to be a degree of apathy, an acceptance of what is doled out and sometimes a degree of gratitude that they are getting anything at all"* (Voluntary agency)

Consultation in these cases could, in actuality, be a matter of the patient agreeing to all suggestions made. One occupational therapist had observed the following conversation in a recent discharge planning meeting;

> *"I went to one (meeting) last week and it was (consultant) 'Right, so, day centre, yes?' and the patient says 'I've been there but I didn't really like it', 'Well, you'll have another try won't you?'. And, this is the CPN, 'And I'll come and visit you next week, yes?' and the patient is saying 'yeah, yeah, see you next week'"*

Elderly people were felt to have particular difficulties in expressing an opinion about their aftercare. This was both because dementia could make informed participation almost impossible and because, as a group, the elderly were felt less likely to disagree with what was proposed. Here carers played a key part in the consultation process speaking on behalf of the patient. Where there was no carer the keyworker may take on this role.

> *"Many patients suffer from moderate to severe dementia and there is a lot of confusion. So, while we try to involve all of them in the care plan, we are also conscious of the fact that sometimes it is not practical because of the nature of the difficulties. But all of the care plans are discussed not just with patient but with their relatives as well... I have always worked on the basis that relatives must be involved... I make a point of inviting relatives to come, in their own time, to come and discuss their care with me, come to ward rounds, come to the review - that's the principle of good practice as far as I'm concerned"* (Consultant, EMI)

There was a belief amongst some patients and carers that they did not have the right to disagree or put forward an opinion.

> *"I don't want to appear too demanding because I'm just a patient"*

> *"The opinion that we have gathered is that P is a long term patient and she is a nuisance and we are carers of P and if we kick up anything about P then we are a nuisance as well. This is the impression that we have been getting all along the line from the psychiatrist to the social worker to the occupational therapist"*

Seeking patients' and carers' consent

There was some debate as to whether patients should be formally asked whether they wanted an aftercare plan. In one area this was a criterion for inclusion into CPA. Opinions on the issue varied from those who believed that it was the patient's right to opt out and their decision should be accepted....

> *"Its their life and its ultimately their choice whether they take up what is proposed or not"* (Voluntary agency)

... to those who felt that people most needing aftercare were the most likely to opt out of it and should be followed up where possible. In reality patients did opt-out, even when they were not formally given this option, by not complying with the plans made.

Even if consultation did not take place, patients were usually asked whether they were in agreement with the plans made. The patient's wishes or agreement were to be recorded on the CPA forms in two areas. In the third area, one ward had begun to get the forms signed by patients to say that they had seen and understood the plans.

It was acknowledged that patients did not always want relatives involved and their wishes were taken into account.

Information for patients and carers

It was believed to be unnecessary to explain CPA as a policy to patients and carers. In two areas, however, it was intended that a leaflet be designed explaining patients' rights to aftercare. There was support for this from many staff. Some more assertive users and carers also expressed a wish to know what their rights were.

> *"If you imagine yourself sitting in a multi-disciplinary meeting discussing with so many people and you have an illness to cope with and you can't remember a thing - but with a booklet you can reflect, go back and read about it and think about it and then you are more able to demand your needs. In a meeting sometimes you are too frightened, there are medical students sitting there whom you don't know"* (CPN)

In all areas, patients were to be made aware of the details of their own personal plan. In two areas it was intended that patients and carers were given written copies of the care plan. This did not appear to happen consistently, however, as very few patients interviewed had a written copy of their plan, particularly if they had been discharged from an acute ward. In the third area patients were made aware of arrangements for individual parts of the plan, rather than the plan as a whole (unless they were under care management).

> *"We will discuss what is being arranged. They need to know about what the arrangement is; 'Here are your tablets, here is your discharge prescription, you can either let the porter get it and it will take you six hours or you can go down to the pharmacy yourself and save yourself a couple of hours'. They know what they have got, the instructions are on the bottles. Similarly if they are going to come to a clinic they have to get an appointment card so they have got the information there, they know they are supposed to be coming. If they are coming to day hospital they are given a timetable - these are the days you are supposed to be coming here and you're coming under your own steam or transport will be provided. So they know. They are not given a piece of paper which says this is your package. They are given the individual bits loose rather than in a bag... It doesn't seem necessary to write it out again in yet another format"* (Consultant, acute)

The nature of the illness and/or the drugs taken for it often made it difficult for patients to remember what took place at aftercare meetings. They were frequently vague about who was present and what was decided.

> *"I was just there, I don't think I was involved at all really. I guess people just turned round and said 'Is that alright?'"* (Ex-patient)

After they had been discharged and the care plan had begun to be put into effect, some ex-patients had little awareness about what was going to happen and were surprised to find a CPN or social worker turning up to visit them. They did not recall this being arranged in advance. Written information that they could read in their own time could help to address this issue. The key information to convey here would be;

- General information about rights to aftercare and how aftercare planning works. For example, explaining that they will be invited to meetings to discuss the care plan, that they are entitled to have their say and so on.

- Names, roles and contact details of keyworker and others involved with care.

- Details of the care plan itself and review dates.

Impact of CPA on the involvement of patients and carers

On the whole, CPA was felt to have made little difference to the extent to which patients and carers participated in the process. There were, however, a few exceptions to this. For example, in one acute unit, CPA was seen to be challenging traditional views on patient involvement and a number of professionals here reported that patients were more involved than previously. The process was now felt to be more collaborative and patients were able to give feedback on what they wanted.

> "Care programme approach is beginning to challenge people about involving patients in the decisions about their care. In some areas where I have worked before it has not been a priority, the consultant ruled more or less and the patient was told what was going to happen. Certainly in teams less efficient and forward looking than (X ward) it is beginning to challenge the more orthodox old-fashioned consultants into beginning to consult with the patients they are caring for" (Health service manager)

In another area patients were also reported as being consulted more than they had been before CPA was implemented. Patients were now felt to be able to make informed choices. In the past they had attended a ward round, been seen by the doctor for a few minutes and then been discussed by those attending afterwards.

Some of the users and carers themselves had found that they were involved in discharge planning to a greater extent than previously. Others, however, experienced no change. It was difficult to gauge the impact of CPA here, however, as factors such as comparison of unlike hospital admissions (for example in different health authorities or to different units) clouded the issue.

7.3   *Involvement of Voluntary Agencies*

All of the voluntary agencies interviewed felt that they had a contribution to make in discharge planning for some patients, especially where;

- They had been in contact with the patient for some time and had built up knowledge of their history and condition.

- They were going to be providing services for the patient after they had been discharged.

- They had specialist knowledge of a relevant field, for example temporary accommodation.

> *"If someone is on a recognised circuit of homelessness .... salvation army, hostels...the likelihood is that we know them anyway and have a lot of experience with them, or we are going to know them soon. Therefore it is not unreasonable for us to be involved in imparting information for those who are planning discharge. Not for us to say you can't do that or you can't do this, but to point out the pitfalls of some accommodation or what happens when accommodation breaks down."* (Voluntary agency)

- There was a need for them to play an advocate role.

The role of voluntary agencies in the CPA procedure was not fully defined in any of the areas, apart from the general consensus that a wide range of people should be involved in discharge planning. In one area it had been suggested that workers from one of the voluntary agencies may take on a keyworker role. However, this had not been possible due to a lack of resources.

Workers from voluntary groups were already involved, to some extent, in attending ward rounds or discharge planning meetings. Sometimes, however, they were not invited when they felt that they should have been. Involvement here gave them much greater appreciation of the care plan as a whole than they would have had if the case had been referred to them.

> *"You have a better chance to know the person, you have a fuller picture of the individual and the package of care that is being discussed for that individual. You have a much fuller picture of what else is available or is perhaps on offer for the individual to make their choices. I think it is helpful to be able to see the individual against this backdrop and be a party to the discussion rather than just have a referral form with various details."* (Voluntary agency)

The voluntary agencies expressed a willingness, in principle, to be involved further. For example, in taking part in more discharge planning meetings or acting as keyworkers. However there were concerns as to what the resource implications of this would be in terms of;

- Staff time needed to attend meetings.

- Staff time needed to fulfil a keyworker role.

- Demand on other resources, such as accommodation or drop-in centres.

7.4 Summary

Collaboration between Statutory Agency Staff

- For CPA to work effectively collaboration was necessary between

  - Ground level staff from health and social services.

  - Statutory agency staff and users and carers.

  - Statutory agency staff and voluntary agencies.

- Multi-disciplinary meetings were usually attended by the patient, the consultant and/or other doctors and ward staff. In many cases CPNs, social workers and relatives would also attend. Occupational therapists, psychologists, day hospital staff, voluntary agencies, housing department staff and GPs were less likely to be involved.

- Multi-disciplinary meetings usually took place in ward rounds. Attendance was generally felt to be useful and more emphasis now placed on aftercare planning.

- Attending ward rounds was time consuming, especially for community staff who needed to travel. There were often competing demands for time, for example social workers may not be working exclusively with people with mental illness. There were further difficulties where wards and community teams were not sectorised in the same manner. Attending ward rounds was easier where there was a set timetable or where separate meetings were held with key people.

- The number of people involved could make meetings difficult to convene. In addition, some professionals were reluctant to be involved.

- Communication was very important in making sure that all involved were aware of the time and place of meetings. Good communication required:

  - The consultant and/or ward staff being aware of parties already involved with the patient.

  - Efficiency in inviting people to meetings.

  - Giving sufficient notice of meetings to allow people to attend.

  - Informing people when meetings had been cancelled or were not running on time.

- Consultants and/or ward staff usually decided who should be invited to multi-disciplinary meetings and some selectivity was in operation here.

- Where a relevant person could not/did not attend a meeting or was not invited there were a number of methods through which they could be involved. For example, the meeting could be postponed or a copy of the outcome sent to them. Sometimes, however, no consultation took place.

- Multi-disciplinary working was easier when:

    - There were good links between the hospital and community services.

    - There were good links between the various staff working in the community.

    - All professionals involved were working or meeting together in one place.

    - The multi-disciplinary team was self contained with a defined client group and aims.

- In one area a "link worker" system had been established to facilitate better communication between the hospital and the community. Here community staff attended ward rounds on a rotation basis and gave feedback to the CMHT. This system ensured that a keyworker was appointed and everyone kept informed.

Involving Users and Carers

- There was widespread agreement with the concept of involving users and carers in CPA and this principle had been incorporated into policy documents.

- The forum for consultation was generally a ward round. Sometimes users and carers were not involved here as:

    - The nature of the illness prevented it.

    - They were not invited.

    - They did not wish to attend or the patient did not wish the carer to attend.

- There was the potential for users and carers to be actively involved in formulating their care plan ie contributing their wishes and opinions. However, this did not always happen because:

    - Ward rounds were perceived as daunting.

    - Patients were afraid to disagree with professionals in case they were not allowed to go home.

    - The nature of the mental illness or the perception that, as a patient or carer, they had few rights to contribute, prevented it.

- Some alternative strategies had been put forward to allow users and carers more scope for participation:

    - Reducing the number of people present at meetings

- Consultation with the keyworker on a one to one basis

- Participating through voluntary sector advocates

- Even where patients were not consulted about their wishes, their agreement to a suggested care plan was often sought.

- At present little information was given to users and carers concerning aftercare, although there were plans to address this. Written information was needed as it was sometimes difficult for users and carers to remember what had been decided at meetings. Ideally this would include:

  - General information about rights to aftercare and the aftercare planning process.

  - Names, roles and contact details of the keyworker and other contributors to the care plan.

  - Details of the care plan itself.

- On the whole CPA was felt to have made little difference to the level to which users and carers were involved. To some extent, however, it was seen to be challenging traditional views on patient involvement and engendering a more collaborative process.

Voluntary Agencies

- Voluntary agencies felt that they had a contribution to make to discharge planning; attending multi-disciplinary meetings, providing services, taking on an advocacy role and acting as keyworkers. They were already involved to some extent, although not as keyworkers.

- Although voluntary agencies were willing to become further involved, the resource implications of doing so would be an important consideration.

CHAPTER 8 Monitoring

In all areas forms had been designed to record information for CPA such as the name and contact details of the patient and keyworker, the care plan, review dates and cases of unmet demand for services. This information was important for use in both providing care programmes on an individual basis and, in aggregated form, in strategic planning.

8.1 The Purpose of Monitoring

In addition to providing a written record of the care plan and identity of the keyworker and others involved with the patient, the information collected also had the potential to be used by managers for a number of purposes;

Monitoring CPA implementation

*   Establishing which patients are receiving CPA, providing evidence of groups which may be "slipping through the net" and groups remaining in hospital due to a lack of community resources.

*   Making sure that CPA procedures are followed properly in hospital eg forms are being filled in and meetings happening

*   Auditing the quality of service, both in the hospital;

    "I am very keen to make sure that CPA is not just a piece of legislation which has come here and is a fad - it is here to stay and should be audited, I feel. If I am not doing my job right I am very keen to make sure that it is picked up and looked at and highlighted otherwise it might as well not be here" (Ward Manager, EMI)

and in the community;

    "At the moment it is a bit like sending a message in a bottle into the sea, nothing comes back. The system is so chaotic out there (in the community), the further it gets away from the hospital the more lost it becomes. Nothing ever gets back to us, so the efforts that you make at the stage of planning discharge soon get dissipated. It doesn't pay out any dividends" (Consultant)

*   Gauging which professions are more likely to be appointed keyworker and the level of resources needed to fulfil this role.

*   Checking whether consistent decisions are made.

Identifying areas where resources are lacking

Records of unmet need could be collated to gauge the type and level of resources needed. There was some concern that unmet need was not being recorded when the assessment was being made. For example, sometimes known deficits in community services were not being highlighted through this process. One manager suspected that people were reluctant to record unmet need lest they be held liable for not delivering a complete service. In other cases unmet need went unrecorded as people were not considered for discharge, for example, because there was no suitable accommodation for them to go to.

One rehabilitation unit had instigated a system for recording unmet need in the past but found that motivation was lacking;

> *"People felt that they were just writing things to go off into the ether - its very difficult for grass roots clinical people to keep writing things that are negative and can't be supplied"* (Health service manager)

Feeding information back to staff

The need to make the information gathered and collated as part of CPA available to staff was recognised. As well as keeping them informed of the overall picture this was also expected to give them incentive to complete paperwork. It was pointed out that form filling could create resistance and that it was essential to give feedback to counter this.

> *"They (discharge plans) are being done and they are being monitored (within our unit) and they are being transferred to a register. OK there are problems with GPs and other agencies not turning up, but they are done and it would be a shame to waste our hard work getting it off the ground if no-one is going to be monitoring it and making use of the information on it. Who is going to be the person to sit down and work through the plans and see why this is happening?"* (Medical Records Officer)

Where staff were aware that information was not being collated, motivation to record it could diminish.

> *"The idea was that we would look at the vulnerable patients and put down the services that the patients required if we could provide them and also the services that we couldn't provide. But is there really any point in me putting down something we can't provide, like the day hospital or the day centre, if it is going to sit in a file? It is not going into the computer as we were told"* (Ward Manager)

8.2 *Implementation of Monitoring*

> *"My greatest concern is that… it was all going to be wonderful when the monitoring was in place but there is no monitoring"* (Social services manager)

Monitoring was felt, at both management and operational levels, to be an essential element of CPA. There were several calls for it to be fully implemented. As yet, however, none of the areas was comprehensively collecting CPA information at a central point, collating it and feeding it back to management or staff. A number of moves had, however, been made in this direction.

- In one area, computerised monitoring of information relating to patients referred to the case management system was being established. This system had the capacity to prompt reviews but had not been extended to include CPA patients as well. In addition, unmet need was recorded and instances gathered at a central point and followed up. The research nurse here had also monitored the completion of CPA paperwork, using a sample of cases on each ward. This was part of the nursing audit.

- In another health authority a psychologist had been monitoring on all wards since April 1992. He had designed a monitoring form, to be completed by ward staff, asking for information such as the profession of the keyworker and whether the client and/or relatives were present. This monitoring had not proved very fruitful due to a lack of information recorded on the discharge and aftercare forms.

  A social work manager in the same area had also carried out some monitoring herself, through her secretary, in order to be able to report on CPA implementation to her managers.

  The generic CPN team here also kept their own records of the discharge planning meetings that they had attended, and these included information on the notice given for the meeting and who attended. This was being collected for the purpose of feeding into central monitoring when established. At another hospital site, copies of CPA paperwork were kept together in folders or box files at various points in the service.

  The CPA forms themselves in this area were kept in the patients' notes and a copy sent to central records. Several staff who had attempted to find aggregated information found this very difficult;

  > "Unless I go now and pick up 50 files of clients who have been discharged and see that they have got a forum and who attended that forum, whether forms went out to invite X,Y and Z, I have no way of knowing that, of the 500+ patients who have come in that we have had 250 or 495 done"

- In the third area, monitoring had initially been carried out by the development officer responsible for CPA implementation. This post had been vacant for a time and central monitoring had ceased. At one acute ward site, however, the medical records officer collated CPA information and fed it back to senior management on a quarterly basis. She pointed out, however, that this monitoring related to the hospital aspects of CPA only and that she had no way of knowing whether care was actually being delivered in the community. There was a need to take an overview of the whole process.

None of the areas was yet able to provide information relating to the numbers and characteristics of people receiving CPA or the numbers of people remaining in hospital due to a lack of community resources.

8.3 Barriers to Effective Monitoring

Two main resources were highlighted as necessary prerequisites for the full implementation of monitoring; a computerised system and designated staff, with sufficient time, to take on responsibility for monitoring.

Computerisation

All three areas were awaiting the installation of computerised systems in the near future. Monitoring of CPA implementation was only one of the roles to be filled by the new systems, two of which were to cover the whole of the health authority. Thus their installation was a major exercise taking into account a wide variety of needs. The necessity to iron out a number of problems had held back progress to some extent.

Computerised systems were expected to enable managers to make full use of the information gathered through the CPA procedure. They would also be useful in prompting reviews and allowing quick access to information such as the identity of the keyworker for a given patient.

As computerisation was at a very early stage, issues concerning joint records, access, confidentiality and consent had not yet been fully addressed. They were, however, recognised as very important areas and a number of concerns were expressed. For example, the issue of whether systems could be shared between health and social services was potentially very problematic.

> "There is a lot of concern about this because of the fact that social services still believe there are many people who come to them who do not want or need the force of the mental health team... They feel that it would adversely affect people if they thought that by coming to see a social worker they would end up on some joint mental health register" (Health service manager)

In two areas social services already had their own computer system but it was not yet clear whether health and social services systems could or would be integrated.

Worries about keeping information secure and confidential were also voiced. For example, there were concerns as to whether passwords would effectively ensure confidentiality. It was considered potentially dangerous in this regard to share health service records with social services and voluntary agencies. The issue of patients' rights to access records was also raised and required resolving.

In one area, where a computerised system was in operation for care management records, access was coded. CPNs had access only to information about their own caseload and the system could only be used when their manager or clerical staff were present. Acute ward staff did not have access to this system. It was envisaged in another area that a separate list identifying which register a patient was on would be used rather than shared access. Discussions on this, however, were at an early stage.

Computerisation was expected to have resource implications both in terms of the hardware and software required and the staff time needed to become familiar with, and make use of, the systems.

Responsibility for monitoring

It was expected that monitoring on an ongoing basis would take up a considerable amount of a staff member's time. Several professionals were of the opinion that it could not properly be carried out as part of an existing role, for example by the managers of individual areas of the service. In one area, the implementation of monitoring had been delayed as the manager in charge did not have the time to take it on as part of her existing workload and also had very little secretarial support.

Two levels of input were required. Firstly there was a need for someone in senior management to be seen to be in overall charge of the ongoing implementation of CPA. They would provide the level of authority necessary to ensure compliance with the requirements of the monitoring process. Secondly, there was a need for someone to take charge of monitoring permanently, making sure that information was recorded and collated. It was likely that a high level of input would be needed from this person on a daily basis. In one area, for example, the medical records officer visited the wards every day and collected discharge planning forms. If necessary she waited while staff completed them. It was expected that this administrative role would require a full time post, at least initially while systems were established. In one area, monitoring CPA had been made part of an information gathering post, with the backing of the senior manager responsible for CPA.

8.4 Summary

- All areas had developed paperwork to record information generated by the CPA procedures. The information gathered had many potential uses; on an individual basis it served as a written record of the care programme and of the identity of the keyworker and other contributors. On an aggregated basis the information could be used to:

  - Monitor CPA implementation, for example to see whether CPA procedures were being followed and for whom, and to monitor the quality of the service provided.

  - Identify areas where resources were lacking.

  - Provide feedback to staff so that they can be kept informed and motivated.

- Information was not being centrally collated and used for the above purposes in a comprehensive manner in any of the authorities.

However, a number of initiatives had been taken to move in this direction.

- There were two main barriers to the implementation of the monitoring process:

  - *Computerisation.*

    All areas were awaiting the installation of computerised systems in the near future. Once up and running it was expected that these would enable managers to make fuller use of CPA information, prompt reviews and allow quick access to information about individual patients (eg the identity of the keyworker). Issues concerning joint records, access and confidentiality had yet to be fully addressed. Computerisation had resource implications both in terms of the equipment required and staff time needed to become familiar with, and make use of, the systems.

  - *Responsibility for monitoring.*

    Monitoring was expected to take up considerable staff time on an ongoing basis. There was a need for a senior manager to take overall charge of CPA and to lend authority to the monitoring process. In addition, there was a requirement for someone to take charge of monitoring on a day to day basis, making sure that information was recorded and collated. This latter role was considered too time consuming to be easily incorporated into an existing role and some felt that it would require a full time post.

PART III

FACTORS AFFECTING CPA IMPLEMENTATION

CHAPTER 9 Factors Affecting CPA Implementation

The main factors which have influenced the effective implementation of CPA
are drawn together in this final chapter. First, some of the key issues
surrounding the initial implementation are discussed. Then some of the
practices felt to contribute to the smooth running of CPA on a day to
day basis are listed.

9.1 Implementation Issues

Need for lead development

The circular left a large degree of scope for interpretation of CPA on a district
basis. Each individual health authority was working through the same
issues in isolation and this duplication of effort made planning for
implementation all the more time consuming. There was certainly a
need for local implementation, and further prescriptive information
from the Department was not generally felt to be required. However,
some form of lead development could have provided cases studies and
examples of good practice which could have been incorporated where
appropriate. Thus planning time could have been saved and early
difficulties in implementation avoided.

Need for further guidance from the Department

On the whole further guidance on CPA from the Department was not seen as
necessary. While some clarification of the aims and objectives of CPA,
especially in relation to care management and/or Section 117 (Mental
Health Act 1983), would be useful to some ground level staff, they
commonly felt that such information should come from their health
authority. In this way the differences could be explained in the context
of local arrangements. It was clear that information conveyed in
Departmental circulars or white papers did not always filter down to
ground level staff. They could perhaps be better reached through
publications specific to their profession.

Overlap between initiatives

Three Government initiatives; CPA, Section 117 of the Mental Health Act 1983
and care management, were perceived to have roughly similar aims.
Responsibility for their implementation and the groups to whom they
were targeted, however, differed. This had caused considerable
confusion even at management level. It would have been useful if the
manner in which these initiatives were intended to tie in together had
been made more explicit.

Misunderstanding of the complexity of CPA

The information given in the circular on CPA was often interpreted to mean that a complicated multi-disciplinary package of care was required. The concept of a minimal care package, for example an out-patients appointment, was not commonly recognised. Patients who needed such a minimal care package were frequently seen as being outside the CPA. While they may still receive the follow-up care they need, CPA paperwork may not be completed for them and put on a central record. In addition, they could also fall outside the arrangements for keyworking and review.

In some cases, it was reported planning meetings were held with more disciplines present than were necessary for the aftercare of the patient concerned. People attended because they felt that CPA required it, rather than because they were needed, and staff time was wasted. CPA was thus seen as more complex, involved or time consuming than necessary for some patients. It was therefore regarded as over-inclusive in relation to some groups of patients.

Offering in-patient care where there are insufficient resources to meet patients' "minimum needs for treatment in the community"

Little attention appeared to have been paid to this requirement of the circular. Such cases were often not recorded and no definitions of "minimum needs" had been formulated.

There were two main difficulties for health authorities in addressing this aspect of CPA:

1.   Those with a shortage of bed space were forced to discharge patients to make room for those needing admission.

2.   Where there was sufficient bed space, such cases had traditionally remained in hospital until adequate care in the community had been arranged. CPA paperwork would not record that this was happening, however, as it was only used for people who were soon to be discharged.

Further impetus for implementation

Much time and effort had been invested in formulating CPA policy and, in three of the areas, in getting the procedures up and running. The initial focus had been on the hospital side; making sure that meetings happened and that paperwork was filled in. This had been rewarded in that procedures for assessment and discharge planning were now largely in place on acute, rehabilitation and EMI wards and in some other facilities. Both in-patient and community staff were, for the most part, familiar with the procedures and their aims.

Following this initial wave of implementation, however, there often appeared to have been a lull in activity. This left the development of some key aspects of CPA outstanding;

- Establishing and clarifying the keyworker role.

- Establishing procedures for prompting and holding reviews.

- Implementing monitoring systems.

In order for CPA to work effectively these issues need to be addressed. A further boost to implementation is therefore required.

9.2 Making the Care Programme Approach Work

The main elements felt to facilitate the smooth operation of CPA on a day to day basis are set out here. They are drawn from suggestions made for change, examples of good practice and elements felt to be missing or not yet fully developed. This section reflects the concerns of the health authorities and social services departments taking part in the study, as they reached the stage of implementation outlined in the above section. In some cases the issues raised could be addressed by changes in procedure. In others, however, there are resource implications to be considered. Not all of the points made will, of course, be relevant or necessary to every area. This list is not exhaustive and it is intended as a starting point for discussion or evaluation, rather than in any way prescriptive.

Implementation/continuing management of CPA

- Having a "driving force" at senior management level with specific responsibility for overseeing the on-going progress of CPA;

  - Having time to put into ensuring that CPA is working and making sure that information gathered is useful and used for management purposes

  - Having the authority to address issues inhibiting CPA

  - Being seen to be in charge of CPA and as someone to whom staff are accountable in its implementation

- Clerical/administrative resources to oversee the working of CPA on a day to day basis;

  - *To gather together and collate information generated by CPA in a form useful to management and to provide feedback to staff*

  - *To provide training on CPA where necessary and to act as a point of contact to discuss any problems experienced with its day to day running.*

This administrative role could be combined with a wider monitoring function including, for example, information gathered from Section 117 (Mental Health Act 1983) or care management processes.

Assessment and discharge planning

- *Assessment*

    - Short and easily manageable assessment schedules (if in use) seen to reflect the circumstances and abilities of the patient.

    - Early instigation of the assessment process so that discharge planning can take place in good time (rather than just prior to discharge).

- *Quality of plans made*

    - Good awareness amongst staff involved in planning of the range of community services in place and levels of availability. A checklist of services could, for example, be used to prompt planning.

    - Adequate levels of community resources in place, especially appropriate accommodation (also community staff and day hospitals/centres).

    - Early involvement of community staff in the planning process so that there is time to arrange community services before discharge.

- *Forum/meetings*

    A forum for assessment and planning where;

    - there is sufficient time for all present to put forward their views on the care plan.

    - the professions present are the main contributors to the care plan but the meeting is small enough to allow the details of the care plan to be resolved ie people peripheral to care planning are kept to a minimum.

    - each person present has an equal say and the meeting is not dominated by one profession eg a consultant, or by another agenda eg teaching junior medical staff.

    It was often found to be difficult to achieve the above in a ward round situation. Consideration could be given to the logistics of using separate meetings.

- *Paperwork/administration*

    - Staff time or extra staff resources allocated for the administration of CPA paperwork so that this does not impinge on time spent with patients. Ward clerks, for example, could be appointed to address this.

    - Efficient systems in place for completing, duplicating and distributing paperwork so that everyone involved is kept informed.

- *Appointing a keyworker*

  - Efficient systems in place for appointing keyworkers so that this is done quickly and any disputes about who should be the keyworker are resolved.

  - The keyworker role shared amongst appropriate professions rather than one being singled out or relied upon.

  - Clear policies established concerning who can or cannot be a keyworker, for example, carers, voluntary agencies, ward staff.

  - Appointment of keyworkers made only with their knowledge and agreement.

  - Appointment of keyworkers made on the basis of patient need.

  - Flexibility built into the keyworker role so that this can be transferred between professions as the patient's needs change.

Delivering the care plan in the community

- *The role of the keyworker*

  - Clear definition of the keyworker role, the level of responsibility implied and the ways in which it differs from existing community staff roles. Establishing to what extent keyworkers will play a co-ordinating role and what level of authority they will have to make sure that care from other sources is delivered.

  - Contact made by keyworkers with the ward and patient prior to the finalisation of the care plan, to get to know the patient and their needs.

  - Consideration given to keyworker staff resources so that they are maintained at a level where they can provide adequate follow-up to individual clients for as long as required.

  - Arrangements made to keep in touch with patients. For example, to follow-up cases where patients do not keep appointments.

  - Mechanisms in place for the various professions involved to keep each other informed about the progress of the care plan.

  - Attention paid to the continuity of care as the client moves between in-patient and out-patient status and vice versa.

- *Reviewing the care plan*

  - Computerised/manual systems in place for prompting reviews.

  - Systems in place for convening reviews eg establishing who is responsible, venue, timing, forum (ie whether there should be a multi-disciplinary meeting), communication etc.

- Recognition of the time needed by keyworkers, consultants and others involved to convene and hold reviews.

- Specific policies in place governing if and when a client should be discharged from CPA.

Working together

- *Collaboration between statutory agency staff*

   - Ground level staff meet face to face to discuss assessment and care planning and keep the relevant professions informed as the patient moves out into the community.

   - Strategies in place to allow professionals involved to participate in multi-disciplinary discussions, for example;

   Holding meetings at convenient locations

   Giving priority to attending such meetings

   Sectorising hospital services to equate with community areas

   Having set timetables for meetings or holding separate meetings when it is possible for people to attend

   Using a "link worker" or similar system.

   - Strategies in place for consulting and informing relevant parties who are unable to attend meetings. For example by sending copies of forms through the post, postponing meetings until a later date or making provisional care plans.

   - Strategies in place for establishing which community services are involved with a patient who has been admitted to hospital. For example, by having key people to contact or by keeping this information on computerised records.

   - Invitation to meetings carried out efficiently, consistently and with enough notice given. Mechanisms in place for informing those involved when meetings have been cancelled or are running late.

   - Good communication between the hospital and community staff, for example, forums for meeting together and involvement of community staff when clients are in-patients, promoting awareness by hospital staff of community services, encouraging dialogue between hospital and community staff.

   - Community staff based together in teams and at the same geographical location.

- *Involving users and carers*

  - Users and carers involved in discharge planning as far as possible ie attending meetings, being consulted about their wishes, giving their agreement to the plans made.

  - Consideration given to alternative forums for consultation to ward rounds. For example, asking the patient how many professionals they would like to have present, the keyworker meeting with patient on one to one basis to seek their views and then feeding them back to the meeting, voluntary agencies playing a role as advocates.

  - Written information provided for users and carers, for example a leaflet explaining rights to aftercare and a copy of care plan together with the contact details for key professionals.

- *Involving voluntary agencies*

  - Clarification of the role of voluntary agencies in CPA.

  - Voluntary agencies involved where appropriate.

Monitoring

- *Collection and collation of CPA information to provide feedback to management and staff.*

  - Establishing which patients are receiving CPA.

  - Ensuring that CPA procedures are followed.

  - Auditing the quality of service, both in the hospital and in the community.

  - Identifying areas where resources are lacking.

- *Implementation of computerised systems to process such information.*

  - Issues around confidentiality, access, consent and joint records resolved.

  - Resources allocated for the necessary hardware and software

- *Staff time allocated*

  - To oversee monitoring and to gather information on an ongoing basis both at management and clerical level

  - To learn to become familiar with and make use of computer systems

9.3 Conclusions

In addition to establishing systematic arrangements for assessing health and social care and ensuring that the relevant services are provided, the care programme approach initiative has acted as a catalyst for discussion and evaluation of a wide range of related issues. These include multi-disciplinary and inter-agency working, the role of users, carers and voluntary agencies, the impact of the organisation of health services (for example sectorisation) on discharge planning and the role of computerised information systems.

The implementation of CPA has involved substantial input from health authorities and social services departments. Implementation has been easier where the foundations of good multi-disciplinary working, strong links between the hospital and the community, effective inter-agency working and other aspects of good practice were already in existence. Where this has not been the case, attention has needed to be given to these issues alongside the establishment of CPA procedures.

Three of the four health authorities involved in the study were well on the way to the full implementation of CPA. A great deal of time and effort had been invested, from health and social services staff at all levels, in establishing the necessary procedures. A further phase of implementation was now needed to ensure that CPA was carried out, on an ongoing and systematic basis, for all those coming into contact with the specialist psychiatric services.

APPENDIX A

SAMPLE AND METHODOLOGY

1. Sample

A total of 169 people took part in the study, of whom 33 gave their views both at stage one and at stage two.

Health authority staff

Senior management (eg mental health unit managers, directorate managers, senior nurse managers, community services managers)	21
Managers of teams/units etc (eg rehab unit, acute unit, CMHT, resettlement team)	4
Policy development officers	3
Consultants (covering acute, rehabilitation and EMI services)	14
Other doctors (acute wards and day hospital)	2
Ward managers (from acute elderly, mother and baby and resettlement services)	9
Ward staff (including ward clerks)	5
Medical records officers/research nurse	4
Occupational therapists (from acute, EMI, rehabilitation, care management, day hospital services)	6
Clinical Psychologists	4
CPNs (from acute, rehabilitation/resettlement projects, EMI and care management services)	19
Total health authority staff	91

Social services staff

Senior managers	16
Team leaders	8
Hospital based social workers	6
Community based social workers (from generic, acute, elderly, care managers, special projects eg mother and baby, resettlement and rehabilitation)	12
Total social services staff	42

Voluntary sector staff (from 4 agencies)	5
Users and Carers[1]	
Users	11
Carers	7
User groups	
MIND user group	4
General user group[2]	8
GP	1
Total voluntary agencies, users and carers, GPs	*36*
Total interviewees	**169**

[1] A total of 16 cases (in two cases both the patient and carer were interviewed).

- 10 female patients and 6 male patients
- 7 patients under 40 years old and 9 patients 40 years or over
- A range of mental illnesses were represented including manic depression, paranoia, senile dementia and schizophrenia.

[2] A user group comprising both users and voluntary sector workers

2. *Selection and Approach*

Interviews with statutory agency staff

The four authorities taking part in the study were selected by the Department of Health to represent diversity in terms of geographical location, co-terminousity with social services departments, type of catchment area and history of psychiatric services. Each health authority and the related social services departments (seven in total) were then approached through a letter to the chief executive of the health authortity and director of social services to seek their agreement to participate. All agreed to take part and provided names of key people within their authority to act as an main point of contact. These were all senior managers with responsibility for mental health services and most had involvement with the implementation of CPA.

Meetings were then arranged with these professionals with the purpose of gathering background information about the services provided for people with mental illness and an outline of the progress of CPA implementation. Also at these initial meetings other key professionals, especially consultants and others involved in developing and implementing CPA policy, were identified. They were then contacted by letter and interviews arranged.

At stage two of the study a further meeting was held with each of the main contact people. Here the progress of CPA since the first phase of the research was discussed and advice was sought on potential interviewees, both at management and operational level. Second interviews were then arranged with the majority of those who had taken part in the first phase. Through these contacts, most of which were at managerial level, arrangements were made to interview staff at operational level[1]. The scope of the study did not, however, allow for ground level staff to be interviewed in all areas of the service in each area. Therefore some selectivity was necessary. Staff working with acute patients, both in hospital and in the community, were included in each area but those working with the elderly or in rehabilitation/long stay facilities were only represented in two of the areas.

Interviews with voluntary agencies

The voluntary agencies involved in the study were those which had been the most closely involved with CPA implementation. They were selected following the advice of the senior health and social services staff responsible for implementation. An approach was made by letter explaining the study which was followed up by a *telephone call* to arrange an interview.

Interviews with users and carers

Interviews with patients who had recently been discharged from hospital under CPA and/or their carers were carried out to find out to what extent they had been involved in care planning and to gain an appreciation of how individual care plans were operating. Mental health services users and their carers were contacted through three sources; consultants, voluntary agencies and user groups.

Consultants were asked whether they would be willing to write to a small number of patients (or their carers where appropriate) to seek their participation in the study. A letter was drafted by S.C.P.R, to be sent out on health authority letterhead, outlining the purpose of the research and asking patients to reply saying whether they would or would not be willing to take part.

In addition, a set of guidelines to be used in selecting suitable patients were drawn up. The main criteria were that patients should have been discharged from hospital using CPA procedures, approximately half should be female and half male, with a spread of ages (half under 40 years and half 40 years or over). A range of psychiatric conditions should be included as well as both voluntary and sectioned patients. However, as each consultant was asked only to contact a small number of patients (typically three or four), the extent to which these criteria

---

1 In one area interviews with one key person from the health authority and one from social services established that implementation had not progressed past the policy stage and thus no further interviews were arranged here.

could be applied was very limited and they served as a rough guideline only.

In three of the areas it was necessary to approach an ethics committee for approval to interview patients. This process was put into motion at phase one and permission was given to seek the participation of patients in each area by the time the second phase commenced.

Although most of the consultants were willing, in principle, to assist with this aspect of the study, contacting patients through this method was not without difficulties. Busy workloads meant that consultants did not always have time to send letters out and, when they did, a number of patients did not reply or declined to take part. These difficulties were addressed to some extent by delegating the selection and contacting of patients to community staff and by supplementing the information in the letter with a personal approach.

In one area a voluntary agency approached a small number of carers of patients who had recently been discharged from hospital to seek their participation in the research. In addition users who belonged to organised groups, for example MIND, were interviewed in two group discussions. These participants had not necessarily been in hospital recently but were able to give a more general view on the CPA concept.

Users and carers taking part in the study were each given £10 in appreciation of their input.

3. *Interviewing*

Interviews with staff at management level generally took place on an individual basis, although, when appropriate and convenient, two or three professionals were sometimes interviewed together. Interviews with staff at operational level were organised with the aim of fitting into busy schedules. Where groups of staff met together, for example in a social work team meeting, it was sometimes possible for the research to be timetabled into the meetings. In other cases small groups of staff were able to meet together to give their views. Usually only one profession was involved in the same discussion so that each staff group would feel able to freely express their own point of view. A total of 57 individual interviews, 12 interviews with two people and 12 discussions with between three and eight people took place.

Interviews with health authority, social services and voluntary agency staff were conducted at the respondent's place of work and generally lasted between 45 minutes and one and a half hours. Often the time which could be made available for interviews, particularly amongst staff at operational levels, was limited by the demands of work. Interviews with users and carers took place within their own homes with the exception of one patient who chose to be interviewed at a day hospital.

114

4. *Analysis and Reporting*

Interviews were tape recorded and detailed notes made using a broad
thematic framework. This allowed the major themes and issues to be
distilled and incorporated into a written report. An interim report was
prepared following the first phase of the study and the issues raised at
that time are now incorporated in this final report. Discussions of the
findings took place with the Department following stage one and a
formal presentation was given to the Department at the end of the
study.

APPENDIX B

TOPIC GUIDES

Topic Guides

Care Programme Approach - Stage Two
Topic Guide for Staff (including Consultants)

1. *Involvement in Planning Implementation Since First Interview (where relevant)*

- progress with planning and implementation in authority as a whole (their awareness of)

- involvement with planning process eg attending working groups, discussions with other staff etc

2. *Extent of Implementation in their Area of Work (cover for different aspects of service with which person is involved eg acute wards, out-patients)*

- To what extent is CPA working on a day to day basis for their patients?

- WHO is included?- criteria used for inclusion? rationale for this?
  - patchiness within wards, certain parts of service included? why?
  - who makes the decision?
  - short stay patients/patients discharging themselves
  - patients opting out of CPA?

- What forums/procedures are used for assessment? formulating a plan of care? eg ward rounds, other meetings, extent to which process is multi-disciplinary, reasons for chosen approach?

- What paperwork is completed? by whom? (use original policy to check)

- Arrangements following discharge

  * are keyworkers appointed? from what profession/s? how is keyworker role allocated? what is their role? reasons for this?

  * review dates set? meetings/consultations held? arrangements for keeping in touch with patients?

- involvement of patients

  agreement to CPA sought (both to being involved and to plans made)
  information given eg rights of patient, copy of plan
  wishes taken into account
(also cover for carers)

- involvement of voluntary agencies and GPs (changes here?)

- if CPA (as described in policy) is not in place probe on procedures for care following discharge from hospital/when in contact with service (ie if already an out-patient/in contact with CMHT)

  - do they view existing procedures as constituting CPA?

  - do they view eg an out-patient appointment with a consultant and subsequent follow-up appointments with him/her as constituting CPA or is it something more involved than this? (emphasis placed on multi-disciplinary working)

3. Implications of CPA

For Staff

- how much has practice changed? whose role has been most affected? how? why?

  * hospital based staff eg extra workloads of ward staff in arranging meetings/liaising/filling in forms, logistics for OTs etc in attending meetings

  * community based staff eg implications for CPNs, SWs and others of being pointed keyworker (time involved, authority/status) and attending meetings.

- have some staff become more involved in discharge planning than they were previous to CPA (or less)

- implications for workloads, ways of dealing with this/implications of it

- need for further training, what type, how provided

- issues to do with attending ward rounds/meetings, strategies to improve this

- changes in multi-disciplinary working

For Patients

- has CPA changed outcome for individual cases being considered for discharge? how and why?

  * changes to discharge decisions eg keeping people in hospital where resources aren't available in the community

  * changes to quality of aftercare received

  * changes in numbers of people "slipping through the net"

  * changes to level of patient involvement in decision making process

For Management

- Use of information collected for management purposes eg monitoring unmet need, monitoring quality discharge planning, guaging resource implications, future plans

- opinions of usefulness of this

- resource implications eg staff time taken to carry out CPA, extra community resources identified as needed and plans to deal with these

4. Factors Affecting the Implementation of CPA

At Organisational Level

eg lack of a driving force at management level, restructuring etc

At Ward/Department/Unit Level

ie why are some wards/departments doing better than others eg attitudes of consultants/other staff, existing multi-disciplinary working

At Individual Patient Level

eg is selectivity meaning that some are missing out on CPA, effects of resource levels in the community to meet individual patients' needs

5. Anonymised Case Studies

Ask R to illustrate some of points made above with case studies - one example of CPA working well and one not working well/not working at all

PROBE ON: background to case eg psychiatric condition, length of stay in hosp., history history of admissions, age, family circs.

process of - deciding to discharge (did resources play a part in the decision?)
- planning aftercare (who was involved? involvement of patient and carer, consideration of their opinions)
- care after discharge (appointment of keyworker, their role, keeping in touch with the patient, reviewing progress)

outcome - Rs satisfaction with care package operating, feedback from patient re their satisfaction
- readmission?

6. In Summary

Main advantages and disadvantages of CPA from their point of view

R's opinion of/attitude towards CPA (as practiced in their authority)

     *   also awareness of opinions of other staff (eg in their team)

     *   opinion/awareness of CPA vs care management

(also ask how more info on CPA from Dept should be communicated ie through what channels to reach R.)

Care Programme Approach
Topic Guide for Patients and Carers

- A research study looking at the sorts of arrangements that are made for people after they leave hospital
- For the Department of Health to assist them in future planning
- Stress confidentiality and anonymity

1. Background

- age, marital status, dependents

Accommodation

- type eg house/flat/bedsit/hostel etc, size, renting/ownership/other
- length of residence
- household/unit composition
- practical help received at home eg housekeeping, shopping

Daytime Activity

- employment - nature of, length of time in present job, how obtained (if since illness), previous employment.
- full time education - nature and length of course, plans for the future.
- unemployment - length of, last employment, why left, job search
- usual daytime activities (if not in full time employment/education) - how is time spent typically
- daytime services (eg day centres, community/youth centres, leisure/sports centres, individual therapy/workshops, social centres/clubs, drop-in centres, libraries etc) - how long used? awareness and use of services provided, how came to start using, if stopped using service/not using service; why?

Social Support/Contact

- personal/social contact - usual extent of contact with other people during the daytime, social activities, emotional support/companionship
- leisure activities - organised and other

Income

- sources; work, benefits, other
- level

Mental Illness

- nature of condition/illness, history of condition, history of treatment i.e time spent as in-patient, number of periods of hospitalisation

```
**         feelings about/satisfaction with
**         changes in situation eg due to illness/since leaving hospital
**         preferences/changes wanted
```

2. Help and Support Currently Received

- are they seeing * consultant/other psychiatrist
  * CPNs/other nurses
  * OTs
  * psychologists/psychotherapists
  * other health service staff
  * social workers/other social services staff
  * their GP
- where and how often do they see each
- what help do they receive from each
- have they had any contact with MIND, NSF or other voluntary agencies

```
** feelings about/satisfaction with
** changes in situation eg due to illness/since leaving hospital
** preferences/changes wanted
```

3. Discharge Planning when last in Hospital

- when were they last in hospital, why was this, was this admission voluntary or did they have to go in?, how long were they in hospital

i) Discharge Decision

- how was it decided that they should leave hospital? what was taken into consideration? eg their state of health, whether there were services available for them in the community?
- were they involved in the discussion and/or decision? to what extent?
- who else was involved eg consultant, ward nurse, community nurse, social worker, voluntary agencies, carer
- satisfaction with how the decision was made (especially the extent to which they, and/or their carer were involved and when they were discharged)

ii) Aftercare Planning

- while they were in hospital were any plans/arrangements made for help and support after leaving hospital

- what were these plans/arrangements; how closely did they meet their needs
- how were they made? meetings, discussions
- were they involved in discussions and decision making? how?
- were they asked whether they wanted these plans made?
- who else was involved? how? (Role of GP)
- at what stage in hospital stay were plans made?
- how did they find out about the plans? were they given a copy of them?
- do they know if information is kept about them and these plans in the hospital? what information? how is it kept? eg computer, were they told about the information kept, was their permission asked?

iii) Aftercare Provided

- what happened after they left hospital; did they receive the services/help arranged? - were there any gaps when services/help were not provided as planned
- do they have any one person overseeing their care now that they are out of hospital/acting as a point of contact eg a keyworker/care manager? what role does this person play?

iv) Reviewing the Care Plan

- since they left hospital, has their care been reviewed
- when and how did this take place eg a meeting
- how, if at all, were they involved?
- who else was involved? how?
- what was the outcome of this? any changes

** feelings about/satisfaction with

** changes in situation eg due to illness/since leaving hospital

** preferences/changes wanted

---

v) Comparison with Previous Discharges from Hospital

- have they noticed any differences in planning or provision of care recently <<before and after CPA implementation>>
- have they been readmitted to hospital since CPA? could better provision in the community have prevented this?

4. Overall Satisfaction with Planning of Discharge and Aftercare

- satisfaction with aftercare provided in relation to perceived needs
- comparison with other experiences of discharge from hospital, both before and after CPA implementation

- knowledge of CPA as a policy and opinions of
- feelings about being included in CPA
- suggestions for change in relation to CPA

Printed in the United Kingdom for HMSO.
Dd.0301678, C3, 11/95, 3400, 5673, 337996.